Gut Health Breakthrough

Resolve Persistent Health Challenges, Autoimmune Disease & Fatigue By Restoring Your Microbiome-A Comprehensive Science-Backed How-To Guide to Heal Inflammation & Feel Better

Keryn Gold, PhD, MBA

Lead With Gold

Author: Keryn Gold, PhD, MBA
Publisher: Lead With Gold, LLC

Legal Disclaimer

This publication is intended to provide accurate and authoritative information regarding the subject matter covered. However, it is sold with the understanding that neither the author nor the publisher is engaged in rendering legal, financial, investment, medical, accounting, or other professional services.

While every effort has been made to ensure the accuracy and completeness of the information in this book, the author and publisher make no guarantees, express or implied, regarding its applicability, reliability, or effectiveness for your individual circumstances. The strategies and advice herein may not be suitable for all individuals or organizations. Readers should seek professional guidance where appropriate.

Neither the publisher nor the author shall be held liable for any direct, indirect, incidental, consequential, or other damages arising from the use or reliance on this book's content, including but not limited to financial loss, legal disputes, or personal and professional consequences.

Responsibility & Risk

By reading this book, you acknowledge that:

- You are solely responsible for your decisions, actions, and outcomes.
- The author and publisher do not accept liability for any financial, legal, or business results based on the material provided.
- Any case studies, examples, and statistics are either drawn from publicly available data or represent composite stories from the author's clients and experience to protect confidentiality.

Legal Notice

Paperback ISBN: 978-1-967456-22-2
Hardcover ISBN: 978-1-967456-23-9
eBook ISBN: 978-1-967456-21-5
Printed in the United States of America
First Edition, 2025
LeadWithGold.com

CONTENTS

Introduction: When the Tests Say "Normal" But You Don't Feel Okay — Why the Hidden World of Your Gut Microbiome Holds the Missing Puzzle Piece for Chronic Pain and Fatigue 1

1. A New Perspective on Chronic Pain and Mystery Illnesses — When the Pain Feels Endless: Could the Answer Lie in Your Gut? 3
2. The Gut–Brain–Immune Axis: Why Your Midsection Matters — How Millions of Microbes Orchestrate Your Body's Pain and Protection 9
3. Lessons from Real Lives: When Healing the Gut Heals Everything Else — The Power of Microbiome Transformations—Stories of Hope and Recovery 17
4. Anatomy of a Comprehensive Gut Analysis: The Roadmap to Root-Cause Insights — Peering into the Hidden Universe Inside You 23

5. Which Test Is Right for You? Comparing Leading Microbiome Panels 29
— From DIY Kits to Advanced Clinical Labs—Finding the Best Fit for Your Journey

6. Why Focusing on Your Microbiome Succeeds Where Others Fail 38
— Pinpointing the True Source of Pain for Lasting Relief

7. Common Conditions Rooted in Gut Imbalances (and How Fixing Them Transforms Health) 43
— Autoimmune Diseases, Chronic Pain, Mood Swings—All Roads Lead Back to the Gut

8. The Intracellular Micronutrient Deficiencies Connection: Intersection With Gut Health 50
— Bridging the Gap Between Nutrient Status and Imbalanced Gut for Deeper Healing

9. Putting It All Together: Your Personalized Action Plan 59
— A 4-Step Strategy to Rebuild, Restore, and Reclaim Your Life

10. FAQs, Pitfalls, and Encouragement 67
— Addressing Doubts, Avoiding Common Mistakes, and Celebrating Small Wins

11. Beware the Traps: Overdoing Probiotics, Selecting the Wrong Strains, and Staying Scam-Free 73
— Safeguarding Your Gut-Healing Journey with Informed Choices

12. Closing the Door on "Mysterious" Pain: Embrace Lasting Relief 80
— Empowering You To Step Confidently Into a Pain-Free Future

Conclusion: Reclaiming Control Over Your Health 85
— How Your Microbiome Empowers You to Break Free from Chronic Pain

Appendix: Therapeutic Doses of Absorbable Micronutrients 90
— How to Support Gut Health With Vitamins & Minerals Your Body Can Actually Use

References 115

Introduction: When the Tests Say "Normal" But You Don't Feel Okay

— Why the Hidden World of Your Gut Microbiome Holds the Missing Puzzle Piece for Chronic Pain and Fatigue

Imagine waking up every morning stiff with pain, reaching for over-the-counter medications that only dull the edges of your discomfort. You've visited countless specialists, tried a dozen different diets, and still, doctors shrug at your normal test results. The message is clear—traditional medicine can't find anything wrong, so maybe you just have to live like this. Except... you don't.

A bold new frontier of research has revealed a hidden world inside each of us—a vast ecosystem of microbes in our gut that do far more than digest meals. These tiny organisms form a living "control center," influencing pain signals, immune function, even our mood. When your gut's delicate balance is disrupted, the resulting inflammation and miscommunication can ripple throughout your body, sparking chronic pain and unexplained symptoms from migraines to extreme fatigue.

What if the true key to feeling like yourself again lies in identifying and correcting these invisible imbalances? What if a targeted stool test, a refined approach to probiotics, or a gut-healing protocol could succeed where years of doctor visits have failed? That's the radical promise of this new science—and it's no exaggeration to say it's changing lives.

This book is your roadmap to a life with less pain and more energy, even if you've almost given up hope. Backed by clinical research and through compelling stories of real people who found relief by healing their microbiomes, you'll see why "mysterious" illnesses aren't necessarily so mysterious after all. We'll explore modern gut-testing technology, investigate why most mainstream medical workups miss crucial clues, and walk step by step through a proven process to rebuild digestive health from the ground up.

Just as important, we'll address what can go wrong—why not all probiotics are created equal, how over-enthusiastic supplement regimens can backfire, and the red flags that help you steer clear of gut-health scams. Knowledge is power, and as you learn exactly how your gut works, you'll be better equipped to spot (and avoid) "miracle cure" scams and fake one-size-fits-all fixes.

Maybe you've been told, "It's just stress," or "There's no explanation for your pain." This book proposes a different story—one that recognizes the gut as an often-overlooked epicenter of chronic symptoms. By the final chapters, you'll have a concrete plan and the confidence to set real change in motion. Healing is possible. You can feel good again. And with the right approach to your microbiome, you might finally unlock the relief you've been searching for all along.

1

A New Perspective on Chronic Pain and Mystery Illnesses

—*When the Pain Feels Endless: Could the Answer Lie in Your Gut?*

Few experiences are more frustrating than persistent pain that lacks a clear explanation. You may have lost count of all the physicians you've visited—rheumatologists, neurologists, pain specialists—and yet every blood test, MRI, or X-ray seems inconclusive. Meanwhile, the unrelenting ache, tension, or fatigue keeps intruding on your day-to-day life. You might feel isolated, or worse, wonder if you're the only one going through this. But you're not alone, and—contrary to what you may have been told—there are legitimate biological underpinnings that can explain the symptoms doctors haven't yet managed to decipher.

The Growing Recognition of "Invisible" Conditions

Traditionally, if pain didn't show up on standard tests, doctors would label it "idiopathic" (meaning "of unknown cause") or suggest it might be "stress-related." While psychological factors can certainly amplify discomfort, new research reveals that the underlying triggers of pain are often physiological—just not in the places most doctors are accustomed to looking. A large and rapidly expanding body of evidence points to the gut microbiome as a hidden driver of persistent, puzzling symptoms, from fibromyalgia to migraines to autoimmune flares.

When Conventional Medicine Falls Short

Consider the typical journey of a chronic pain sufferer:

1. **Primary Care Checkups**
   - You might start with a general practitioner, who runs basic blood tests looking for markers of inflammation or infection. If nothing flags, the physician may recommend over-the-counter anti-inflammatories or physical therapy.
2. **Referrals to Specialists**
   - Next come the specialists. A rheumatologist rules out rheumatoid arthritis or lupus, a neurologist checks for nerve compression or multiple sclerosis. If scans show no physical damage, you're often told "there's nothing structurally wrong."
3. **Symptom Management**
   - In the absence of a clear diagnosis, symptom management prevails—prescriptions for stronger painkillers or antidepressants. Meanwhile, the actual cause of your pain remains unexamined.

This cycle can go on for years. Yet in multiple peer-reviewed studies, patients eventually found relief once they tackled the health of their intestinal tract—whether that meant eliminating overgrowths of harmful bacteria, balancing intracellular micronutrients, resolving gut permeability ("leaky gut"), or replenishing beneficial flora that produce anti-inflammatory compounds.

Why the Gut Matters More Than You Think

It may sound odd at first: **why would the microbes in your colon have anything to do with pain in your back, shoulders, or head?** The key is understanding the gut's role as a control center for systemic inflammation, immune regulation, and even neurological function. Here's how it can happen:

1. **Inflammatory Spillover**
    - When the gut microbiome is imbalanced—too many inflammatory bacteria, not enough beneficial species—these microbes can release toxins into the bloodstream. This process, sometimes aided by increased intestinal permeability, triggers chronic, body-wide inflammation.
2. **Immune System Confusion**
    - The gut is home to over 70% of your immune cells. If these cells are constantly bombarded by microbial stress signals, they can become "hyper-vigilant," attacking not just pathogens but also healthy tissues. Autoimmune flares, joint pain, and generalized aches can emerge or worsen.
3. **Nervous System Cross-Talk**
    - The vagus nerve and other neuronal pathways connect the gut to the brain. Disruptions in gut flora can alter neurotransmitter production—serotonin, GABA, and more—exacerbating pain sensitivity and mood disturbances.

Put simply, an unhealthy gut "primes" the body for inflammation and heightened pain signaling. Correcting dysbiosis—an imbalance in gut bacteria—has been shown to reduce markers of systemic inflammation, improve mood, and lower overall pain levels in many controlled clinical trials.

Embracing a Systems-Based Mindset

One of the biggest shifts happening in modern medicine is the move toward a **systems-based** perspective. Rather than treating the body as a collection of isolated parts, more clinicians and researchers recognize that the gut, brain, and immune system are constantly in communication. This integrated view is precisely why chronic pain might not originate at the site of pain itself, but rather in the signals that your gut microbiome sends (or fails to send). This is also why Fascial Counterstrain, and resolving Intracellular Micronutrient deficiencies, as outlined in my other books, are gaining increased traction, as they approach health challenges systemically and focus on addressing the root cause, rather than just masking isolated symptoms.

A Real-World Example

Imagine a patient with severe fibromyalgia, experiencing diffuse muscle and joint pain without a definitive lab result to explain why. Traditional assessments show no obvious tissue damage or nerve compression. Yet a gut microbiome test might reveal profoundly low levels of butyrate-producing bacteria—a deficiency that correlates with higher inflammatory markers in her bloodstream. When she adopts a microbiome-healing regimen (incorporating prebiotic fibers, targeted probiotics, and an anti-inflammatory diet), her pain scores drop significantly (Castro et al., *Journal of Translational Medicine*, 2022). None of this would show up on an X-ray or standard blood test, but the link is backed by peer-reviewed research and the patient's tangible improvement.

Putting the Pieces Together

Chronic pain and mysterious symptoms aren't necessarily locked in your genetic fate—nor do they always demand indefinite rounds of medication. Instead, they can often be traced to **invisible** imbalances in the gut or the inability to properly absorb key nutrients. This first chapter aims to set the stage for a bold, evidence-based claim: **addressing your microbiome can drastically improve—and sometimes fully resolve—unexplained pain and long-standing health issues.**

- **No, it's not a cure-all**: Every individual is different, and some conditions do require conventional interventions. But addressing the gut frequently provides the missing puzzle piece for many conditions long deemed "idiopathic."

- **Yes, the science is real**: Ongoing clinical studies and systematic reviews document improvements in everything from chronic fatigue syndrome to IBS once gut imbalances are corrected.

Preview: Where Do We Go Next?

In the chapters that follow, you'll learn how your gut, brain, and immune system communicate—a surprisingly intricate dance that either fosters health or feeds pain. You'll discover the methods doctors and functional medicine practitioners use to **analyze** your gut microbes, including next-generation sequencing and advanced stool testing. Real-life recovery stories will show you how a gut-centered approach can be transformative, even for people who've felt hopeless for years.

For now, rest assured there is a logical, biologically sound explanation for what you've been enduring. The fact that previous doctors didn't fully understand where to look for it doesn't make it any less real. As you keep reading, you'll gain the tools to take action—developing a scientifically grounded plan to mend your gut, ease your pain, and reclaim your health and vitality.

Key Takeaways

- Chronic pain often persists when traditional tests don't reveal an obvious cause.
- A growing body of peer-reviewed research links gut imbalances (dysbiosis, leaky gut) to widespread inflammation and neuropathic pain.
- Embracing a systems-based approach—viewing the gut, immune system, and brain as interconnected—unlocks new avenues for lasting relief.
- Evidence shows that restoring the gut's microbial balance can improve fibromyalgia, chronic fatigue, migraines, and other "mysterious" conditions once considered largely "untreatable."

You may have thought, "It just has to be this way." Science begs to differ. The next chapters will open up a world of possibilities that current medical paradigms often overlook—possibilities that just might change how you feel, forever.

2

The Gut–Brain–Immune Axis: Why Your Midsection Matters

— How Millions of Microbes Orchestrate Your Body's Pain and Protection

When you think about "gut health," you might picture digestion—nutrients absorbed, waste excreted, maybe a little bloating or indigestion here and there. But beneath the surface, your gastrointestinal tract does so much more. A thriving community of microorganisms—bacteria, fungi, even viruses—lives in your gut and actively communicates with the rest of your body, notably your brain and immune system. This three-way conversation, often called the **gut–brain–immune axis**, helps determine everything from how you process emotions to whether your joints ache in the morning. Understanding how these systems interact reveals why seemingly isolated symptoms—chronic pain, anxiety, autoimmune flare-ups—can all stem from imbalances in your gut.

1. The "Forgotten Organ" in Your Belly

Scientists have dubbed the gut microbiome our "forgotten organ" because it operates almost like a distinct entity within our bodies. Together, the trillions of microbes in your intestines weigh roughly as much as your brain (around three pounds) and contribute over eight million unique genes—far more than the human genome itself. These genes help regulate:

- **Metabolism** – Certain microbes break down dietary fiber into short-chain fatty acids like butyrate, which not only fuel your colon cells but also have potent anti-inflammatory effects throughout your body.

- **Immune Function** – A well-balanced microbiome teaches immune cells which particles are harmless and which ones warrant attack.

- **Neurological Pathways** – Gut microbes produce or stimulate the production of neurotransmitters (serotonin, GABA) that affect mood, stress resilience, and pain perception.

In short, gut bacteria do much more than help digest food; they form a dynamic network that touches nearly every bodily system.

2. The Gut–Brain Dialogue: More Than a One-Way Street

We often talk about "gut feelings," but the connection between belly and brain goes beyond metaphor. The **vagus nerve**—a bidirectional highway of neurons—runs from your brainstem to multiple organs, including the gastrointestinal tract. Through this nerve, microbes in your gut can send chemical signals that influence mood, cognition, and **pain sensitivity**.

How Gut Signals Affect Your Brain

1. **Neurotransmitter Production**
    - Many gut bacteria synthesize molecules like GABA, dopamine, and serotonin. While these neurotransmitters don't all cross the blood-brain barrier directly, they can stimulate neural pathways or immune cells that do communicate with the brain.
2. **Immune Modulation**
    - Chemical messengers (cytokines) released by immune cells in the gut travel through the bloodstream to the brain, affecting inflammation and possibly triggering or dampening pain signals.
3. **Stress and Cortisol**
    - Chronic stress disrupts the gut lining, making your microbiome more prone to imbalance (dysbiosis). In turn, dysbiosis can heighten stress responses by sending alarm signals to the central nervous system.

This continuous conversation explains why mental health challenges like depression or anxiety sometimes improve when gut health is addressed—and why chronic pain can be exacerbated by emotional stress.

3. The Immune Connection: Training Your Defenders

Your gut is not just a digestive tube; it's also the largest immune organ in the body. Around 70% of your immune cells reside along the intestinal lining.

These cells learn to differentiate between friend and foe by interacting with gut microbes. When the microbiome is well-balanced:

- **Regulatory T-Cells Are Cultivated**
    - Beneficial bacteria can encourage the production of regulatory T-cells, which help prevent the immune system from attacking the body's own tissues.
- **Harmful Invaders Are Kept in Check**
    - Pathogenic microbes struggle to gain a foothold when beneficial species are abundant, because "good" bacteria outcompete them for space and resources.

But if the microbiome skews towards harmful or inflammatory strains—due to poor diet, chronic stress, or antibiotics—your immune cells can overreact, targeting not only intruders but also healthy tissue. This overzealous inflammation can present as joint pain, skin rashes, or autoimmune conditions (Fasano, *Physiological Reviews*, 2020).

4. Chronic Inflammation: The Common Denominator

When gut dysbiosis persists, low-grade inflammation often becomes chronic. Lipopolysaccharides (LPS)—toxic components on the outer membrane of certain bacteria—can leak from your gut into circulation. The immune system interprets them as a call to arms, unleashing inflammatory cytokines that can sensitize nerve pathways and amplify pain signals.

Systemic Ripple Effects

- **Joint and Muscle Pain**
    - Long-term inflammation can heighten pain receptors or wors-

en autoimmune arthritic processes.

- **Mood Swings and Fatigue**
    - Inflammatory signals crossing the blood-brain barrier can disrupt neurotransmission, contributing to fatigue or depressive symptoms.
- **Heightened Pain Perception**
    - Pro-inflammatory chemicals may lower your threshold for pain, turning mild discomfort into debilitating episodes.

Thus, an imbalanced gut can push your body into an inflammatory loop that exacerbates pain and ignites mysterious ailments other tests fail to catch.

5. Real-World Illustrations: When Healing the Axis Heals the Body

- **Case: Migraines Linked to Dysbiosis**
    - A study in *mSystems* found that individuals prone to migraines often have higher levels of nitrate-reducing bacteria in the mouth and gut. These bacteria can overproduce nitric oxide, a known migraine trigger. Patients who corrected this imbalance with targeted probiotics and dietary adjustments saw a reduction in migraine frequency.
- **Case: Autoimmune Relief through Probiotic Strains**
    - In a clinical trial focusing on rheumatoid arthritis, participants taking a specific strain of *Lactobacillus* reported less morning stiffness and fewer tender joints than those on placebo. Researchers theorized that reducing gut-driven inflammation

lowered the overall autoimmune burden.

- **Case: Psychological Wellness and the Gut**
    - A double-blind study revealed that supplementing with certain *Bifidobacterium* strains for eight weeks improved stress-related GI symptoms and even reduced participants' perceived anxiety. This underscores the gut-brain link in real, measurable outcomes.

6. Putting It All Together: The Holistic Power of the Gut–Brain–Immune Axis

The takeaway? Your gut, brain, and immune system form an interconnected triad, constantly exchanging information and adapting based on the microbial environment in your intestines. When that environment is balanced, your body can excel at self-regulation—keeping inflammation in check, modulating pain signals, and supporting robust mental and emotional health. Conversely, when the microbiome tilts toward dysbiosis, the entire system becomes more reactive, fueling persistent pain and fatigue that mystify conventional diagnostics.

By uncovering and correcting imbalances—through comprehensive stool analysis, targeted probiotics, dietary shifts, and lifestyle practices that nurture beneficial bacteria—you stand a better chance of reducing your pain at its source. In the next chapters, we'll explore exactly how to investigate your gut microbiome, interpret results, and implement personalized strategies that heal the axis at each of its crucial junctions. If you've ever wondered why a single pill rarely solves chronic conditions, the answer lies right here: **the gut–brain–immune axis** is as intricate as it is powerful, and harnessing its benefits demands an informed, systemic approach.

Key Insights

1. **The Gut Microbiome Is a Powerhouse**
    - Far from merely aiding digestion, it heavily influences inflammation, immunity, and even neurotransmitter activity.
2. **Communication Flows in All Directions**
    - Signals move from gut to brain (and back) through neural, hormonal, and immune pathways. Disrupt one link, and the entire system can suffer.
3. **Low-Grade Inflammation Amplifies Pain**
    - Chronic exposure to microbial toxins (LPS) and inflammatory cytokines lowers the threshold for pain and triggers autoimmune responses.
4. **Balancing the Axis Can Relieve Chronic Conditions**
    - Evidence from clinical trials shows that shifting the gut's microbial balance can reduce migraines, joint pain, and even anxiety.
5. **Next Steps: Testing & Targeted Interventions**
    - Subsequent chapters will detail how to test your gut microbiome and build a personalized blueprint for restoring gut–brain–immune harmony.

If you've spent years trying to explain to doctors how you can "just feel" something is off, science now confirms your instincts: the gut is both a command center and an early warning system. Healing it might just be the single most impactful move you can make to resolve pain and protect yourself against a host of chronic health challenges.

3

Lessons from Real Lives: When Healing the Gut Heals Everything Else

—The Power of Microbiome Transformations—Stories of Hope and Recovery

For all the scientific explanations and research studies that point to our gut microbiome as a cornerstone of health, the human stories are powerful reminders of the impact gut health can have on real lives. There's a growing community of individuals who've experienced dramatic turnarounds simply by focusing on the balance of microbes in their digestive tract. These transformations aren't fleeting or "one in a million"—they're being documented in medical case studies, clinical trials, and patient forums worldwide. In this chapter, we'll dive into a few compelling narratives that illustrate how resolving hidden gut issues can release people from years of chronic pain and persistent ailments that had defied every other intervention.

1. Fibromyalgia: A Subtle Shift That Changed Everything

Fibromyalgia is infamous for its elusive nature—patients endure widespread pain, fatigue, and cognitive "fog," yet standard diagnostic tests rarely reveal a concrete cause. Many sufferers bounce from one specialist to another, trying painkillers, antidepressants, or gentle exercise regimens with limited success. But a 2024 clinical trial offered a groundbreaking alternative: fecal microbiota transplantation (FMT). Researchers took gut bacteria from healthy donors and transferred it to participants with fibromyalgia. Astonishingly, most participants reported a marked reduction in pain within weeks. Follow-ups at six and twelve months showed sustained improvement in pain scores, energy levels, and mental clarity. What changed wasn't just a single "miracle microbe," but an entire microbial ecosystem—one that reduced inflammatory signals and restored better communication between the gut and nervous system. While FMT remains a relatively new therapy, the outcomes strongly suggest that balancing gut flora can be the missing link for certain fibromyalgia patients.

2. Chronic Fatigue Syndrome (ME/CFS): Unlocking "Remission Events"

Myalgic encephalomyelitis, more commonly referred to as Chronic Fatigue Syndrome (ME/CFS), has long baffled doctors. Patients are often bedbound or at best severely limited in daily activities. A breakthrough occurred when two individuals, each diagnosed with ME/CFS for over a decade, experienced what they called "remission events" after tackling a bacterial infection. When they were prescribed broad-spectrum antibiotics for an unrelated illness, their longstanding symptoms abruptly lifted. It seemed counterintuitive—antibiotics typically don't improve ME/CFS—but both patients then took high-dose probiotics to replenish their gut microbiome. Something about the "reboot" effect led to sustained energy, reduced pain, and better mental focus for months afterward. While not everyone with ME/CFS would replicate these exact circumstances, the story underscores how rebalancing the gut might be a catalyst for remission in conditions once thought untreatable. Indeed, larger clinical studies are now investigating fecal transplants in ME/CFS, hoping to replicate these surprising outcomes under controlled conditions.

3. Autoimmune Arthritis: When Meds Fail and Microbes Prevail

Autoimmune forms of arthritis, such as rheumatoid arthritis (RA) or ankylosing spondylitis (AS), cause severe joint or spinal pain. Standard treatment often involves immunosuppressive drugs or biologics designed to tamp down the body's overactive immune response. These medications can be effective, but they also carry substantial risks and sometimes fail entirely. In one striking case, a patient with extremely aggressive AS tried multiple high-end drugs with no relief. Desperate for another option, he underwent a series of three FMT procedures. Within weeks of the first transplant, both his spinal pain and gastrointestinal inflammation started to improve. After completing all three, he achieved a stability and comfort level he hadn't known in years. Lab markers also reflected a decrease in systemic inflammation. Doctors speculated that the healthy microbes introduced via FMT recalibrated his immune system, mitigating the persistent inflammatory assault on his spine. While this is just one case, it aligns with other reports suggesting that a targeted correction of gut dysbiosis can significantly impact autoimmune activity.

4. IBS and Other Digestive Disorders: Surprising Revelations

Sometimes the most dramatic results are found exactly where you'd expect—at the source of gastrointestinal distress. Irritable Bowel Syndrome (IBS), for instance, comes in multiple forms (diarrhea-predominant, constipation-predominant, or a mix), and the symptoms can be debilitating: cramping, bloating, unpredictable bowel habits. Many sufferers embark on strict elimination diets or turn to antispasmodics without lasting relief. Comprehensive stool analyses often reveal stealth issues like methane-producing bacterial overgrowth or high levels of inflammatory markers. Once these are addressed—with a combination of antimicrobial treatments, specialized probiotics, and dietary changes—symptoms frequently diminish. Beyond IBS, similar stories abound for conditions like Crohn's disease and ulcerative colitis, where fecal transplants and microbiome-focused therapies have occasionally led to remission in cases once labeled "untreatable." Although the response varies, it's evident that interventions targeting the gut ecosystem can unlock possibilities far beyond the conventional approach of merely suppressing symptoms.

5. The Bigger Picture: Why These Stories Matter

At first glance, fibromyalgia, ME/CFS, autoimmune arthritis, and IBS might appear to have little in common besides their stubbornness to conventional treatment. Yet in all these examples, the crucial breakthroughs came from realigning the gut microbiome. The underlying logic is straightforward: a well-functioning microbiome helps maintain a robust, yet balanced, immune system, prevents "leaky gut" that allows inflammatory toxins to enter the bloodstream, and fosters healthy gut-brain communication. When any of these components malfunction, it's a recipe for system-wide chaos—a perfect storm of persistent inflammation, hyperactive pain signals, and a body that can't properly repair itself.

These case studies aren't meant to promise overnight cures or to suggest that a single probiotic capsule will fix complex illnesses. They do, however, highlight a paradigm shift: for many people, the gut is where seemingly unrelated issues converge. It's also where remarkable turnarounds can happen when the right steps are taken. Chapter 4 will outline exactly what these "right steps" look like in practice, from lab-based stool analysis to interpreting which specific microbes may be at fault—or in short supply. But for now, let these stories serve as evidence (in addition to the many clinical trials) that balancing gut flora isn't a fringe idea; it's an emerging frontier in legitimate, research-backed medicine that is offering new hope to those who've struggled the longest.

Key Takeaways

1. **Broad Applicability**: Conditions like fibromyalgia, ME/CFS, autoimmune arthritis, and IBS share a hidden link—imbalances in the gut microbiome often play a pivotal role.

2. **FMT as a Case in Point**: Fecal microbiota transplants, while still considered innovative, have delivered dramatic benefits in some cases, underscoring the power of microbial realignment.

3. **Microbiome "Resets"**: Antibiotics or specific probiotics can, under certain circumstances, trigger a meaningful change in gut ecology that leads to unexpected remission events.

4. **Root-Cause Focus**: Resolving the imbalance in gut flora may accomplish what decades of symptomatic treatments could not, offering relief at the source rather than another band-aid solution.

5. **No Guarantees, but Genuine Hope**: While no single therapy works for everyone, these stories underscore the potential and urgency of investigating your gut as a primary target for genuine healing.

The weight of personal testimony combined with increasingly robust science points to one conclusion: a dysfunctional gut can be central to chronic pain and illness, but by the same token, restoring gut health can liberate you from conditions that seemed inescapable. As we move on, you'll see how these stories aren't anomalies; they're previews of what becomes possible when you bring your microbiome back into balance.

4

Anatomy of a Comprehensive Gut Analysis: The Roadmap to Root-Cause Insights

—Peering into the Hidden Universe Inside You

When it comes to identifying the root causes of chronic pain, inflammation, or the many "mystery" symptoms that elude traditional tests, comprehensive gut microbiome analysis is increasingly seen as a game-changer. Unlike a standard stool test that might only check for blood or a specific pathogen, advanced analysis dives into the very DNA of the microbes in your digestive tract. It also measures key markers of digestive function and inflammation. The result is a detailed snapshot of how well—or poorly—your gut is functioning as an ecosystem. In this chapter, you'll learn what a truly thorough gut evaluation looks like and why it can be transformative for those dealing with persistent health issues.

1. The Basics: How a Stool Sample Reveals Your Inner Landscape

Most comprehensive tests begin with a stool sample you collect at home. Kits typically include a small container and preservative solution. Though it may sound off-putting, these kits are designed to make collection as straightforward as possible. Once the sample reaches the lab, technicians and automated systems perform a series of analyses to identify the types of microorganisms present and assess markers of gut health. One vital concept is that multiple methods (culture, PCR, DNA sequencing, microscopy) may be used in tandem. For example, some labs culture a portion of the sample to see which bacteria or yeasts grow under specific conditions, while others run polymerase chain reaction (PCR) tests to detect targeted pathogens. More advanced panels employ next-generation DNA sequencing—allowing them to identify microbes (including hard-to-culture species) in astonishing detail.

2. Mapping the Microbes: 16S vs. Shotgun Metagenomic Sequencing

There are two main DNA-sequencing approaches you'll often hear about. The first is 16S rRNA gene sequencing, which zeroes in on a specific region of bacterial DNA (the 16S rRNA gene) that acts like a "fingerprint" for identifying bacteria at the genus level. It's cost-effective and widely used, but may not always pinpoint the exact species. The second is shotgun metagenomic sequencing. Rather than focusing on one genetic region, shotgun sequencing reads all the DNA in the sample. This allows for more precise identification—sometimes down to bacterial strains—and can detect viruses, fungi, and archaea as well. It's more expensive but yields a richer data set on what each microbe can do (e.g., produce certain vitamins or toxins). Both methods can yield important insights, but if you want the deepest possible dive into your gut's microbial residents, shotgun metagenomics is considered the gold standard.

3. Functional Markers: Beyond Microbial IDs

The best gut tests don't just list what microbes are present; they also measure how well your gut is operating. This includes inflammatory markers like calprotectin, lactoferrin, or secretory IgA, which can reflect ongoing gut-lining inflammation or immune activation. Digestive efficiency markers—such as pancreatic elastase—gauge whether your pancreas is secreting enough enzymes to break down food properly. When enzyme levels are low, undigested nutrients linger in your gut, fueling harmful bacteria and contributing to bloating or malabsorption. Some advanced panels also measure short-chain fatty acids (SCFAs) like butyrate and propionate, which support gut-lining health and provide anti-inflammatory effects. By integrating these data points with microbial identification, you get a clearer picture. You might learn, for example, that you're low in butyrate-producing species while also seeing a spike in pro-inflammatory markers. That's a clear call to action: increase your fiber intake, introduce the right probiotic strains, and calm gut inflammation.

4. Targeted PCR Panels: High Specificity, Limited Scope

Some clinical tests (e.g., GI-MAP) rely heavily on quantitative PCR to detect known pathogens or opportunistic microbes like H. pylori, Candida, or Giardia. PCR is extremely sensitive, making it excellent for catching specific troublemakers that might be behind diarrhea, bloating, or pain. However, if a certain organism isn't on the lab's "watch list," it won't show up. That's why a test combining PCR panels with broader 16S or shotgun metagenomic methods can be invaluable.

5. The Microbial Diversity Factor: Why It Matters for Pain and Immunity

A high diversity of gut microbes—think of it like a thriving rainforest with lots of distinct species—generally correlates with better health outcomes. Conversely, an imbalanced microbiome, dominated by a few inflammatory species, is linked to a range of chronic conditions, from autoimmune diseases to metabolic syndrome. Many comprehensive reports now include a "diversity score" or "dysbiosis index" that helps you instantly see whether your ecosystem is robust or precarious.

6. Key Insights You Can Gain from Comprehensive Testing

A thorough gut test can highlight pathogen overgrowth, revealing if an overabundance of harmful bacteria or a parasitic infection might be fueling chronic pain or fatigue. It can also show if you're deficient in beneficial microbes such as Lactobacillus or Bifidobacterium. Additionally, certain markers may indicate a leaky gut, elevated zonulin, or other signs of intestinal barrier dysfunction. You can even uncover nutrient malabsorption issues that point to the need for pancreatic enzymes or dietary tweaks. Put together, these findings form a blueprint for targeted intervention, whether that means eradicating a bacterial overgrowth, boosting deficient strains, or supporting digestion.

7. Working with Practitioners vs. At-Home Kits

Some test panels are ordered exclusively through healthcare providers, offering in-depth clinical markers. Others can be ordered online without a prescription. While at-home kits (like Viome or Ombre) can provide interesting insights, they often lack thorough pathogen screening or deeper functional markers. If you're grappling with chronic pain or autoimmune issues, a practitioner-ordered test may be more actionable. However, consumer-oriented tests can still be a useful entry point for identifying glaring imbalances.

8. Empowering Your Healing Journey

Having your test results explained by a knowledgeable health professional—one who understands both conventional and functional approaches—can be a turning point. You'll learn which dietary strategies, probiotics, or antimicrobials can directly address the imbalances uncovered. In many cases, just one or two targeted interventions—such as eradicating a bacterial overgrowth or supplementing with butyrate-boosting prebiotics—dramatically eases pain and inflammation. The key is not to treat a gut test as a novelty, but as the first step in a guided transformation. This is especially critical if you've suffered for years without clarity. Comprehensive gut analysis shines a light on previously hidden culprits, giving you a map for true root-cause healing.

Key Takeaways

1. Advanced testing goes beyond "normal" stool checks to identify both the spectrum of your gut flora and the functional markers that point to inflammatory or digestive issues.

2. 16S vs. shotgun sequencing: each has pros and cons, but shotgun often offers deeper insights, especially when paired with functional assessments.

3. Functional markers matter, revealing if your gut is inflamed, leaky, or under-producing key enzymes.

4. Tests can reveal a clear path forward—like targeting a hidden pathogen, boosting beneficial strains, or supporting digestion.

5. Working with a practitioner skilled in interpreting these tests maximizes the odds of meaningful, long-term improvements.

Up next, we'll compare some of the most popular microbiome tests—both at-home and practitioner-ordered—to help you decide where and how to begin your investigation. Armed with knowledge of your personal gut profile, you'll be well on your way to forging a plan that finally relieves persistent pain and puzzling health issues at the source.

5

Which Test Is Right for You? Comparing Leading Microbiome Panels

—From DIY Kits to Advanced Clinical Labs—Finding the Best Fit for Your Journey

You're now aware that a comprehensive gut analysis can reveal hidden contributors to chronic pain, unexplained fatigue, or immune-driven inflammation. But which specific test should you choose? With new microbiome panels hitting the market every month—ranging from simple mail-in kits to sophisticated clinical diagnostics—it can be difficult to know where to start. Some tests aim to personalize lifestyle recommendations, while others home in on pathogens or measure an array of inflammatory markers. In this chapter, we'll review the most common options in both consumer and practitioner-ordered categories, outlining the pros, cons, and likely use cases for each. This guidance will help you select a test aligned with your goals, whether you're simply curious about your gut's overall "health score" or actively seeking the root cause of severe, ongoing symptoms.

1. At-Home Consumer Kits: A First Step into the Microbiome

Many people begin their gut-health journey with direct-to-consumer tests that don't require a doctor's prescription. Often priced between $120 and $400, these kits let you collect a stool sample at home and mail it to the company's lab. Results are then delivered via an online portal or app.

- **Viome**
    - **Method**: Metatranscriptomic sequencing (analyzes microbial RNA)
    - **What You Get**: Personalized "Health Scores" (e.g., gut lining health, inflammatory activity, and microbe diversity), food recommendations, and the option to purchase custom supplements based on your profile.
    - **Pros**: Potentially captures active microbial gene expression, giving a functional snapshot rather than just identifying species present. Provides user-friendly, AI-driven diet suggestions.
    - **Cons**: Proprietary technology makes independent validation difficult. Mostly geared toward wellness and optimization rather than diagnosing pathogens or clinical conditions.
- **BIOHM**
    - **Method**: 16S rRNA sequencing, including both bacteria and fungi.

   - **What You Get**: A "Gut Score," microbial composition breakdown, basic dietary suggestions, focus on fungal balance (unique among many consumer kits).
   - **Pros**: More affordable (often around $130), user-friendly interface, highlights the often-overlooked fungal component.
   - **Cons**: Limited scope for specific pathogens; results can be broad, lacking deeper functional markers like inflammation or enzyme output.
- **Ombre (formerly Thryve)**
   - **Method**: 16S rRNA sequencing.
   - **What You Get**: An app-based report detailing bacterial composition and product recommendations for targeted probiotics.
   - **Pros**: Typically under $150, straightforward process, decent entry-level look at major bacterial groups.
   - **Cons**: No pathogenic screening or advanced inflammation markers; recommendations sometimes lean toward Ombre's own supplement line.
- **Thorne Gut Health Test**
   - **Method**: Metagenomic sequencing in partnership with Onegevity/CosmosID.
   - **What You Get**: Species-level identification, biodiversity scores, diet and supplement recommendations aligned with Thorne products.
   - **Pros**: More comprehensive than 16S, can identify non-bacte-

rial microbes and some functional genetic pathways.

  - **Cons**: Generally more expensive ($190–$200 range), heavily tied to Thorne's supplements.

These DIY tests can offer a baseline snapshot of your gut environment and can be a great starting point for healthier eating and lifestyle changes. However, if you're dealing with chronic or severe symptoms, you may need more in-depth, clinically oriented testing to pinpoint targeted treatment strategies.

2. Practitioner-Ordered Comprehensive Panels: A Deeper Dive

Healthcare professionals, such as functional medicine doctors or integrative nutritionists, often use lab-developed tests that merge advanced microbiome profiling with clinical markers. Prices typically range from $300 to $600 (or more), but the data is far more actionable for serious conditions.

- **GI-MAP (Diagnostic Solutions Laboratory)**
  - **Method**: Quantitative PCR (qPCR) panel screening dozens of bacteria, parasites, fungi, and viruses.
  - **What You Get**: Pathogen detection (like C. difficile, Salmonella, H. pylori), opportunistic microbes, antibiotic resistance genes, plus immune markers like secretory IgA and inflammation markers such as calprotectin.
  - **Pros**: Excellent for identifying specific troublemakers, fast turnaround time, widely used in functional medicine circles.
  - **Cons**: Primarily tests for what's on the panel; doesn't always give a complete picture of all microbes present.

- **GI Effects Comprehensive (Genova Diagnostics)**
    - **Method**: Multi-modal (culture + PCR + microscopic ova & parasite exams + 16S rRNA for select commensals).
    - **What You Get**: Digestion, inflammation, and gut microbiome categories; SCFA levels; a dysbiosis index; pathogen screening.
    - **Pros**: Extremely thorough, measuring digestion markers like pancreatic elastase, metabolic byproducts, and an array of bacteria/yeast.
    - **Cons**: More expensive ($500–$600), results can be somewhat technical to interpret, especially if done without professional guidance.
- **Doctor's Data GI 360**
    - **Method**: Integrates culture, PCR, and next-generation sequencing for 116 microbial targets, plus inflammatory and digestive markers.
    - **What You Get**: A microbiome diversity score, parasites and opportunistic bacteria detection, SCFA levels, and antibiotic sensitivity on cultured organisms.
    - **Pros**: Merges old-school culture (to test antimicrobial sensitivities) with cutting-edge molecular approaches. Offers a broad panel of microbes and functional indicators.
    - **Cons**: Pricey ($450–$500), results can be dense, requiring interpretation from a trained practitioner.
- **Additional Specialty Labs**

 - There are emerging labs using shotgun metagenomics (e.g., CosmosID) or advanced methods for specific conditions (e.g., Parasitology Inc. for thorough parasite checks). Some require direct ordering from a healthcare provider or specialized referral.

Practitioner-based tests usually yield a more comprehensive understanding of your gut's microbial ecosystem along with clues about inflammation, leaky gut, and digestive efficiency. While the cost is higher, the information is often critical for tackling persistent or serious health concerns where quick-fix approaches have failed.

3. How to Decide: Key Factors to Consider

- **Symptom Severity and Complexity**
  - Mild or occasional bloating might be addressed with a budget-friendly consumer kit, while chronic conditions (fibromyalgia, autoimmune disorders) call for in-depth clinical panels.
- **Goal: General Wellness vs. Targeted Intervention**
  - If you just want to optimize your diet and see if you have any glaring microbial imbalances, a DIY kit may suffice. But if you suspect a hidden infection or are managing unexplained pain, a clinically oriented test offers more actionable details.
- **Cost and Insurance**
  - Some labs accept insurance or offer partial reimbursement for practitioner-ordered tests. Direct-to-consumer kits are usually out of pocket but may have promotions or subscription discounts.

- **Interpretation and Support**
    - At-home reports focus on user-friendly insights but rarely include pathogen analysis or medication guidance. A healthcare provider can interpret robust test results in context, discussing potential antimicrobial therapies, prescription medications, or advanced supplements.

4. Red Flags and Caveats

While the microbiome testing field is exciting, it's also brimming with marketing hype. Be cautious of:

- **Overly Simplistic "Miracle" Claims**. A single test or probiotic won't universally fix every health issue.
- **Opaque Methodology**. Reputable labs publish technical details about how they analyze samples. If it's vague or proprietary to the point of secrecy, you won't be able to gauge quality.
- **Subscription Scams**. Some services pressure you into expensive monthly probiotics or supplements. Make sure any ongoing costs align with real, research-backed value.

5. Getting the Most Out of Your Chosen Test

- **Prepare**: Follow your kit's instructions closely—mixing stool with the provided preservative, storing it properly, and mailing it promptly.
- **Time Your Test**: If you've recently finished antibiotics or drastically changed your diet, the timing can affect results. Give your gut a few weeks to stabilize first, unless your practitioner advises otherwise.

- **Plan for Follow-Up**: Testing isn't an end in itself. It's the launchpad for targeted strategies—ranging from dietary adjustments to specific antimicrobials.

- **Consider Retesting**: If you implement a significant gut-healing protocol, you may want to re-check your microbiome in a few months to track progress.

Key Takeaways

1. **Consumer vs. Clinical**: At-home kits offer a snapshot of microbial diversity and wellness tips, while practitioner-ordered tests delve deeper into pathogens, inflammation, and gut function.

2. **Matching Goals to Methods**: Opt for a simple kit if you're generally healthy and curious, or a comprehensive panel if you're dealing with chronic or severe symptoms.

3. **Interpretation Matters**: A complex test is most valuable when paired with an expert who can craft a personalized treatment plan.

4. **Beware the Hype**: The microbiome industry attracts plenty of overstated promises. Look for transparent, scientifically backed testing methods and labs.

5. **Action-Oriented**: Testing is a means to an end—understanding your gut's unique needs so you can move toward lasting relief from pain, inflammation, and related health issues.

In the next chapter, we'll discuss why zeroing in on the microbiome can often produce results where standard treatments have failed—specifically looking at the chain reaction between gut health, immune function, and your body's pain signaling pathways. Armed with the right test and a targeted plan, you'll be set to tackle the root causes of chronic conditions you once felt were incurable.

6

Why Focusing on Your Microbiome Succeeds Where Others Fail

—Pinpointing the True Source of Pain for Lasting Relief

It's one thing to understand the gut's role in overall health, and quite another to appreciate why microbiome-focused therapy so often helps where traditional medical approaches fail. For many patients, addressing diet or stress provides only partial relief—and in worst-case scenarios, they're left with an unending cycle of doctor visits and prescription changes. In this chapter, you'll see why a comprehensive evaluation of gut health often becomes the "missing piece" in the puzzle of chronic pain, persistent inflammation, and confounding symptoms that defy standard treatments.

1. Going Upstream: Tackling Root Causes Instead of Just Symptoms

Conventional healthcare frequently zeroes in on symptom management. You have joint pain? Here's a painkiller. Persistent headaches? Try a migraine medication. Depressed mood alongside pain? Let's add an antidepressant. While these measures can offer temporary respite, they seldom address the hidden biological triggers driving the discomfort.

A microbiome-centered approach, by contrast, probes underlying mechanisms like dysbiosis (an imbalance in gut flora) and leaky gut syndrome. These issues can fuel systemic inflammation, alter immune responses, and distort pain processing in the nervous system. By restoring gut balance, you're effectively turning off the upstream source of that inflammatory cascade—often yielding deeper, more sustained improvements than simply masking symptoms.

2. Viewing the Body as an Interconnected System

A rheumatologist examines joints, a gastroenterologist looks at the GI tract, a neurologist focuses on nerves—yet chronic conditions frequently span multiple body systems. The gut–brain–immune axis ties together these seemingly separate domains. When the gut is dysregulated, it can amplify signals in the immune system and brain, manifesting as chronic pain, brain fog, or psychiatric concerns like anxiety and depression.

By targeting the gut, a microbiome-focused strategy inherently takes a "systems biology" perspective. It doesn't isolate symptoms within a single organ; rather, it recognizes how the gut's ecosystem influences immunity, hormonal regulation, and neural pathways. This holistic stance often reveals the common thread uniting otherwise puzzling or "idiopathic" syndromes, helping practitioners and patients alike see the bigger picture.

3. Personalized Medicine: One Gut Profile Does Not Fit All

Two patients might present with the same condition—say, fibromyalgia or IBS—but have radically different gut imbalances. One could have an overgrowth of methane-producing archaea, contributing to constipation and systemic toxicity; the other might show low levels of butyrate-producing bacteria, fueling inflammation and heightened pain sensitivity. Both individuals are classified under the same condition, yet the specific interventions needed to restore balance vary enormously.

Microbiome testing pinpoints these differences. Rather than one-size-fits-all advice ("take a probiotic; eat more fiber"), treatment becomes individualized: maybe your gut requires antimicrobials for a parasite, or you need a high-butyrate diet, or targeted supplementation to elevate levels of specific Lactobacillus strains. This tailored approach is far likelier to yield real results than generic recommendations, which can fail—or even exacerbate issues—in certain gut environments.

4. The "Invisible" Infections and Imbalances Standard Tests Miss

Healthcare typically runs basic stool checks for acute pathogens (like Salmonella or C. difficile) or blood markers for systemic infections. Chronic overgrowths and subclinical infections often remain undetected by these methods. Comprehensive stool analysis can uncover parasites like Blastocystis, opportunistic fungi like Candida, or subtle bacterial overgrowths that standard panels overlook. Such findings are critical because:

- **Low-Grade Infections** can produce toxins that perpetuate low-level inflammation.
- **Overgrowths** of normally harmless organisms can disrupt nutri-

ent absorption and immune balance.

- **Resistant Strains** may require specific interventions—some respond to herbal antimicrobials, others need targeted antibiotics.

By identifying these hidden culprits, a microbiome-focused plan hits the bullseye. Instead of attributing "mystery" symptoms to psychosomatic or "functional" diagnoses alone, it addresses tangible biological disruptions.

5. Holistic, Long-Term Health vs. Short-Term Suppression

For patients trapped in the loop of acute symptom control, it can feel like whack-a-mole—treat one complaint only for another to flare up. A gut-centered method aims to rebuild a resilient microbiome, which in turn stabilizes immune function, modulates hormonal signals, and improves nutrient metabolism. The net result? Fewer flare-ups across multiple body systems, not just the original complaint that prompted medical consultation. Over time, this can lessen dependency on medications and reduce the likelihood of relapses.

6. When Conventional Therapies Plateau, the Gut May Hold the Key

Consider the patient with rheumatoid arthritis who responds poorly to biologics, or the fibromyalgia sufferer who's tried every pain medication with minimal relief. Investigating and correcting gut dysbiosis can sometimes achieve results that eluded the most advanced pharmaceutical options. Why? Because you're not just blocking pain pathways or suppressing immune activity—you're recalibrating the entire ecosystem that orchestrates inflammation and pain signals.

This is not to discount the importance of mainstream therapies. Often, a blend of conventional and gut-focused interventions is the sweet spot. However, ignoring the microbiome—and the profound systemic influences it exerts—can leave a giant gap in treatment plans for stubborn, hard-to-treat conditions.

Key Takeaways

1. **Root-Cause Power**: Microbiome therapy addresses the upstream triggers of inflammation and pain, offering a deeper fix than symptomatic relief alone.

2. **Whole-System Perspective**: Gut-focused care inherently acknowledges the interplay of digestive, immune, and nervous systems, bridging conventional medical silos.

3. **Personalized Solutions**: Different forms of dysbiosis require tailored interventions—what works for one person's gut may not work for another's.

4. **Uncovering Hidden Imbalances**: Comprehensive stool analysis can reveal low-grade infections, stealth pathogens, or overgrowths that basic tests miss.

5. **Holistic Recovery**: A balanced microbiome not only reduces immediate symptoms but also lowers the risk of future flares, fostering sustained wellness.

Next, we'll explore the myriad conditions—beyond chronic pain—linked to gut imbalances and how restoring microbial harmony can transform health. Whether you struggle with autoimmunity, metabolic issues, or even mood disorders, the microbiome often plays a pivotal role that conventional care might be overlooking.

7

Common Conditions Rooted in Gut Imbalances (and How Fixing Them Transforms Health)

—Autoimmune Diseases, Chronic Pain, Mood Swings—All Roads Lead Back to the Gut

It's easy to think of the gut and its microbes as relevant only for digestion—issues like bloating, gas, or irritable bowel syndrome. But emerging science continues to map unexpected links between dysbiosis (microbial imbalance) and ailments that show up in completely different organ systems. The underlying theme is that **systemic** inflammation and immune misregulation often originate in the gut, even if the eventual symptoms manifest elsewhere, such as your joints, nerves, skin, or brain. This chapter walks through some of the most common conditions associated with gut dysfunction, explaining why rebalancing the microbiome can be a linchpin for genuine, lasting relief.

1. Chronic Pain Syndromes

Fibromyalgia, Migraines, and Beyond

- **Fibromyalgia**
  Characterized by widespread pain, fatigue, and cognitive "fog," fibromyalgia often defies conventional treatments. Dysbiosis can contribute to central sensitization—a hyper-reactivity of the nervous system triggered by chronic inflammatory signals emanating from an unhealthy gut. Research has found distinct gut microbiome profiles in fibromyalgia patients, pointing to disruptions in beneficial bacteria that modulate pain perception. Balancing gut flora with targeted probiotics, dietary changes, or fecal microbiota transplantation (FMT) has shown promise in reducing pain severity and fatigue.

- **Migraines**
  Headaches may seem worlds apart from gut flora, yet studies reveal that migraine sufferers often harbor an overabundance of nitrate-reducing bacteria—microbes capable of producing nitric oxide (known to trigger headaches in some individuals). Migraines can also be exacerbated by systemic inflammation. By taming gut imbalances, people frequently report fewer or less intense migraine episodes, especially when combined with identifying and removing dietary triggers that feed troublesome bacterial strains.

2. Autoimmune Disorders

Rheumatoid Arthritis, Lupus, Multiple Sclerosis, and More

- **Rheumatoid Arthritis (RA)**
  RA involves the immune system attacking joint linings, causing pain, swelling, and potential joint deformities. Multiple studies link an overgrowth of specific gut bacteria—like *Prevotella copri*—to early-stage RA. High levels of pro-inflammatory bacteria can break down the gut barrier, priming the immune system to misfire. Interventions like targeted antimicrobials or probiotic supplements can alter the gut environment, potentially reducing autoimmune flare-ups.

- **Lupus (SLE)**
  While lupus typically manifests with rashes, joint pain, and organ complications, gut permeability and an imbalanced microbiome are increasingly recognized as major drivers. Beneficial bacteria help regulate immune tolerance, whereas harmful ones can prompt the body to attack its own tissues. Some lupus patients experience notable remission of symptoms after improving gut health, highlighting a key therapeutic avenue often overlooked.

- **Multiple Sclerosis (MS)**
  In this neurodegenerative disease, the immune system assaults the protective myelin sheath around nerve fibers. Although MS is centered in the brain and spinal cord, research implicates the gut as a contributor—certain bacteria appear to influence immune cell activity, either exacerbating or calming autoimmune attacks. Clinical trials testing targeted probiotics and FMT are underway, suggesting that addressing dysbiosis could moderate MS flare severity.

3. Metabolic and Cardiovascular Issues

Obesity, Type 2 Diabetes, and Heart Health

- **Obesity & Type 2 Diabetes**

Imbalanced gut flora can increase caloric extraction from food, disrupt hunger hormones, and trigger chronic low-grade inflammation tied to insulin resistance. Studies in both animals and humans show that transplanting a "lean" microbiome can spur weight loss or improve metabolic markers in those with obesity or type 2 diabetes. While these transplants aren't a silver bullet, they underscore the gut's pivotal role in metabolic regulation.

- **Cardiovascular Risk**
  Certain gut bacteria produce trimethylamine N-oxide (TMAO), a compound associated with atherosclerosis and heart disease. Dietary changes that modulate TMAO-producing microbes—or supplementation with probiotics that counteract them—could lower cardiovascular risk. A healthy microbiome also supports optimal cholesterol metabolism and blood pressure regulation.

4. Neurological and Mental Health

Anxiety, Depression, Autism Spectrum, Parkinson's Disease

- **Mood Disorders**
  Roughly 90% of the body's serotonin is produced in the gut. When harmful bacteria outcompete the beneficial species that help synthesize mood-regulating neurotransmitters, conditions like anxiety and depression can worsen. Conversely, introducing psychobiotic strains (probiotics with mental health benefits) can reduce depressive symptoms and lower stress-related inflammation.

- **Autism Spectrum Disorder (ASD)**
  Research suggests many children with ASD have distinct gut microbiota and often struggle with co-occurring digestive issues. Interventions like FMT have shown promise in improving not just GI symptoms but also certain behavioral metrics. While it's

early days, this relationship highlights how gut-based therapies might support neurodevelopmental conditions.

- **Parkinson's Disease**
  Parkinson's primarily affects motor function due to dopamine neuron loss in the brain. Yet gastrointestinal symptoms often precede the neurological decline by years. Some studies propose that abnormal protein aggregates may even start in the gut and travel via the vagus nerve to the brain. By modulating gut microbes, scientists hope to slow disease progression or at least alleviate digestive and inflammatory burdens.

5. Allergies and Skin Conditions

Eczema, Psoriasis, and Food Sensitivities

- **Eczema (Atopic Dermatitis)**
  Imbalances in gut flora can compromise the gut lining, allowing inflammatory compounds to circulate and exacerbating skin flare-ups. Certain probiotic strains have been linked to improved eczema outcomes, likely by regulating immune overreactions and strengthening gut-skin barriers.

- **Psoriasis**
  Characterized by red, scaly patches on the skin, psoriasis is now understood as an immune-mediated disorder with gut connections. Some psoriasis patients show a microbiome profile low in anti-inflammatory bacteria. Clinical anecdotes and pilot studies suggest that correcting dysbiosis can reduce the frequency or intensity of flares.

- **Food Intolerances**
  Not everyone who reacts badly to dairy or gluten has a clinical allergy or celiac disease; many have subclinical sensitivities height-

8

The Intracellular Micronutrient Deficiencies Connection: Intersection With Gut Health

—Bridging the Gap Between Nutrient Status and Imbalanced Gut for Deeper Healing

Invisible gut imbalances can exacerbate chronic symptoms—but so can hidden deficiencies in vitamins, minerals, and other essential nutrients. While these two factors might seem unrelated, the reality is they interact constantly. Your gut microbes depend on a steady supply of micronutrients for their own metabolism, and in turn, their activity (or inactivity) significantly shapes which nutrients you absorb. This chapter explores how dysbiosis (an imbalanced gut) both causes and is caused by micronutrient deficiencies, creating a self-perpetuating loop that can intensify inflammation, fatigue, and susceptibility to disease. Understanding this dual relationship can be the key to more precise, lasting relief.

1. When Gut Dysbiosis Leads to Micronutrient Deficiencies

A healthy microbiome acts almost like another organ, synthesizing vitamins, releasing enzymes that aid mineral absorption, and supporting the integrity of your intestinal lining. But when the microbial balance skews, that beneficial synergy breaks down.

- **Competition and Consumption**
  Some bacteria consume the very nutrients you rely on—like iron or vitamin B12—leaving you with less to absorb. Overgrowths (e.g., SIBO) exacerbate this effect by increasing the sheer number of microbes competing for the same resources.

- **Damage to the Gut Lining**
  Dysbiosis can erode the protective mucus layer or produce toxins that inflame intestinal tissue. This damage impairs the ability of intestinal cells to absorb vitamins and minerals, leading to deficiencies despite an adequate diet.

- **Reduced Vitamin Production**
  Beneficial microbes help produce a range of B vitamins and vitamin K, contributing to your overall reserves. Wiping out these producers—say, via broad-spectrum antibiotics or a long-standing imbalance—shrinks your internal supply.

Key Insight:

- Even if you eat a nutrient-rich diet, a dysfunctional microbiome can sabotage absorption. Meanwhile, ongoing gut inflammation—frequently seen in dysbiosis—further lowers micronutrient levels by impairing intestinal function.

2. How Micronutrient Deficiencies Disrupt Gut Balance

Micronutrients aren't just for you; your gut microbes also depend on them. When you're low on essential minerals or vitamins, your microbial ecosystem may shift toward species better adapted to scarcity or inflammation, often crowding out beneficial strains.

- **Weakening the Barrier**
  Nutrients like zinc and vitamin A are integral to maintaining tight junctions and healthy mucus. Inadequate supplies open the door to "leaky gut," allowing endotoxins or bacteria into the bloodstream and fueling even more inflammation.

- **Immune Dysregulation**
  Vitamins D and C, along with trace elements like selenium and zinc, help shape immune responses in the gut. If these run low, the body's ability to keep harmful microbes in check suffers—dysbiosis proliferates.

- **Selective Pressures**
  Certain bacterial species thrive in nutrient-poor environments where others can't survive. Iron deficiency, for example, may favor microbes adept at scavenging minimal amounts of iron, overshadowing strains that require more robust mineral availability.

Key Insight:

- Micronutrient deficiencies can be an inciting factor for gut imbalances, not merely a byproduct. Restoring adequate nutrient status often paves the way for beneficial microbes to re-establish themselves.

3. Mechanisms Linking Gut Function and Intracellular Nutrient Status

Microbial Enzymes & Nutrient Liberation

Beneficial microbes produce enzymes that unlock minerals bound in plant compounds and synthesize certain vitamins (like folate, biotin, or vitamin K). If these enzymes or microbes are absent, you won't access the full nutritional value of your meals—even if you're technically ingesting enough.

Transporter Proteins & SCFAs

Short-chain fatty acids (SCFAs)—byproducts of microbial fermentation—lower gut pH, improving the solubility of minerals like calcium and magnesium. SCFAs also strengthen intestinal cells, indirectly boosting expression of nutrient transporter proteins. Conversely, pathogens may generate chemicals that hamper absorption or degrade transport proteins.

Immune Inflammation & Hepcidin

When dysbiosis persists, the immune system produces inflammatory cytokines. High levels of these signals induce hepcidin, a hormone that traps iron in storage sites. This "anemia of chronic disease" lowers circulating iron, depriving both you and your microbes of a critical resource.

ent Testing can be done by **SpectraCell, Vibrant America,** or **Genova Diagnostics,** and **measures nutrients inside your cells** that standard blood tests (which just look at the serum) miss. These intracellular micronutrient tests can detect malabsorption and intracellular deficiencies resulting from pharmaceutical use or ingestion of forms your body can't digest or absorb well. I have another book (*The Root Cause of Your Symptoms, Uncovered)* that digs into this topic in detail, outlining the specific most absorbable forms and therapeutic doses of each micronutrient for various conditions and symptoms. A summary list can be found in the Appendix, and additional free and downloadable resources are available at LeadWithGold.com/heal.

2. **Dietary Synergy**
   Opt for nutrient-dense foods that naturally support beneficial microbes: diverse plant fibers, fermented options, lean proteins, and essential fats. Minimizing ultra-refined carbs cuts off "junk fuel" for opportunistic bacteria.

3. **Targeted Supplementation**
   If tests reveal deficiencies, replenishing vitamins or minerals may jump-start gut healing. Correcting zinc deficits, for instance, with the most absorbable forms, tightens the gut barrier and reduces inflammation.

4. **Probiotics & Prebiotics**
   Certain strains help with nutrient absorption; Lactobacillus species can assist with iron or magnesium uptake. Bifidobacterium strains produce B vitamins. Fiber-rich prebiotics feed SCFA-producing microbes.

5. **Address Root Causes**
   Chronic infections, low stomach acid, or autoimmune conditions can sabotage nutrient status. Removing these obstacles helps pre-

vent perpetual micronutrient depletion.

6. **Lifestyle & Stress Management**
Chronic stress disrupts gut barrier function and micronutrient metabolism. Adequate sleep, moderate exercise, and lower stress support a stable gut environment, which, coupled with ingestion of nutrients your body can actually use, ensuring the vitamins and minerals you consume are properly utilized.

Summary and Next Steps

The interplay between gut microbes and intracellular nutrient levels is a two-way street—and a crucial piece of the puzzle in persistent health challenges. Dysbiosis impairs nutrient absorption and can degrade the very vitamins or minerals you rely on. Meanwhile, insufficient micronutrients weaken the gut lining and immune defenses, giving opportunistic microbes a foothold. Much like rebuilding a house from its foundation, overcoming chronic symptoms often demands reinforcing both the gut's microbial community **and** your body's nutrient status at the same time. In the next chapter, where we dive deeper into building a comprehensive healing plan, remember to look beyond single culprits. The synergy—between optimizing your microbiome and replenishing core nutrients—may well be the linchpin that finally moves the needle on long-standing inflammation, fatigue, and pain.

Key Takeaways

1. **Bidirectional Impact**: Dysbiosis can spark vitamin and mineral deficiencies—and vice versa—forming a self-reinforcing loop of malabsorption, inflammation, and microbial imbalances.

2. **Mechanisms Matter**: Microbial enzymes free up nutrients, while micronutrients bolster the gut barrier and immunity.

Deficits on either side disrupt these processes, triggering deeper imbalances.

3. **Chronic Disease Roots**: Autoimmune flares, chronic fatigue, metabolic syndrome, and neurological issues often feature both gut flora disturbances and micronutrient deficits.

4. **Dual-Focused Treatment**: Testing both gut health and nutrient levels, correcting deficiencies, and rebalancing the microbiome collectively yield better outcomes than targeting either factor alone.

5. **Practical Action**: A synergy of diet (fiber-rich, nutrient-dense), strategic supplementation, probiotics, and stress reduction is vital for breaking the cycle of poor gut function and micronutrient depletion.

With this understanding, you're better equipped to build a robust protocol—one that acknowledges not just "what's missing" nutritionally, but also how your gut community influences, and is influenced by, every vitamin and mineral you consume.

- A "synbiotic" combines probiotics and prebiotics for a synergistic effect. For example, a supplement that includes *Bifidobacterium* strains plus inulin or a FOS-based prebiotic can help boost colonization of good microbes more effectively than either component alone.

ip: In certain severe cases (e.g., recurrent *C. difficile* infections or refrac-
ory autoimmune disorders), Fecal Microbiota Transplantation (FMT) nay be considered under medical supervision, providing a broad infusion of healthy donor microbes.

3. Repair: Strengthening the Gut Lining and Calming Inflammation

Even with the right microbes in place, a damaged or "leaky" gut lining can continue to spark systemic inflammation. The Repair phase zeroes in on healing this vital barrier.

- **Key Nutrients for Repair**
    - **L-Glutamine**: An amino acid that supports the integrity of intestinal cells (enterocytes). Often taken as a supplement (5–10 grams daily) to help seal the gut lining.
    - **Zinc Carnosine**: Shown in studies to bolster mucosal defenses and reduce inflammation in the GI tract.
    - **Omega-3 Fatty Acids**: Anti-inflammatory fats found in fish oil or algae-based supplements can reduce overall gut and systemic inflammation.
- **Anti-Inflammatory Agents**
    - **Curcumin** (turmeric extract), **quercetin**, and **aloe vera** are known for their soothing properties within the GI tract. They

9

Putting It All Together: Your Personalized Action Plan

—A 4-Step Strategy to Rebuild, Restore, and Reclaim Your Life

By now, you've seen how chronic pain, autoimmune flare-ups, and stubborn fatigue can trace back to hidden imbalances in the gut. You also know that advanced stool testing can unearth the root issues, from dysbiosis to stealth infections. The question remains: **What do you do about it all?** This chapter lays out a practical, four-step framework to revitalize your microbiome and, in turn, help alleviate long-standing aches, inflammation, and confusing symptoms. These steps—Remove, Repopulate, Repair, and Rebalance—are foundational in functional medicine circles for tackling gut-related problems at their source. Whether you're just starting your journey or have been struggling for years, this plan can serve as a roadmap to genuine healing.

1. Remove: Clearing Out the "Bad Guys" and Irritants

The first step is to eliminate or reduce factors that contribute to dysbiosis and inflammation. This often involves:

- **Pathogen Eradication**
    - If your stool test uncovers a specific bacterial overgrowth, parasitic infection, or fungal colonization, your practitioner may recommend antimicrobial medications or targeted herbs (e.g., oregano oil, berberine, or caprylic acid).
    - Be sure to follow a clinician's guidance regarding dosage and duration, especially if prescription antibiotics or antiparasitics are involved.
- **Dietary Clean-Up**
    - Processed foods, excess sugar, and artificial additives can feed harmful microbes. An elimination diet—removing common irritants—can give your gut a chance to reset.
    - If you have known triggers (such as FODMAPs for IBS, or certain nightshades for autoimmune flares), your stool results can confirm whether these foods are truly problematic or if another culprit is at play.
- **Toxin Reduction**
    - Chronic exposure to alcohol, pesticides, and environmental toxins can degrade gut lining integrity. Minimizing these factors helps reduce the overall inflammatory burden in the gut.

Tip: The "Remove" phase can range from a few weeks to several months, depending on the severity of infections or overgrowths. During this peri-

od, you might notice a temporary shift in symptoms—s
before improving, especially if harmful microbes release t
off.

2. Repopulate: Introducing Beneficial Strain
Strong Foundation

Once the gut environment has been cleared of major disruptive
time to replenish beneficial microbes. This can happen througl

- **Probiotic Supplements**
    - Strain selection matters. For instance, *Lactobacillus rh*
      GG may help reduce certain inflammatory bowel sym
      while *Saccharomyces boulardii* can combat yeast overg
      Your stool test results can guide which strains are most n
    - Look for products with transparent labeling—specific str
      colony-forming units (CFUs), and evidence-based for
      tions.
- **Prebiotics and Fermented Foods**
    - Prebiotics (fibers that feed beneficial bacteria) are fou
      foods like onions, garlic, chicory root, and asparagus. S
      mental prebiotic powders (e.g., inulin, FOS) can also hel
      introduce them slowly to avoid gas or bloating.
    - Fermented foods (kimchi, sauerkraut, kefir) deliver li
      tures and can be easier on the gut compared to higl
      probiotic capsules—though some individuals with seve
      biosis may need to start cautiously.
- **Synbiotic Approaches**

can help reduce discomfort and promote tissue regeneration.

- **Lifestyle Modifications**
    - Chronic stress and poor sleep wreak havoc on gut tight-junction proteins, perpetuating a leaky gut. Incorporating relaxation techniques and prioritizing restorative sleep support deeper healing.

Tip: Track your progress with symptom journals or periodic gut-marker retests (like secretory IgA and zonulin). That helps verify if your gut lining is indeed on the mend.

4. Rebalance: Maintaining a Resilient Microbiome Long-Term

After the initial phases of clearing bad microbes, introducing beneficial ones, and repairing the intestinal lining, the final step is about *sustainability*—ensuring your gut remains an environment where health-supporting microbes can thrive.

- **Diet as a Lifestyle**
    - Return to (or maintain) a varied, nutrient-dense way of eating rich in whole foods, fiber, and minimal ultra-processed ingredients. A Mediterranean-style diet or a plant-forward approach often works well for gut diversity.
    - Continue to limit refined sugars, excess alcohol, and artificial additives that feed dysbiotic organisms.
- **Periodic "Gut Check"**
    - Some individuals benefit from periodic comprehensive stool retesting, especially if they notice relapses in symptoms.

  - Minor adjustments—e.g., temporarily increasing probiotics or focusing on specific fermentable fibers—can keep your microbiome balanced in the face of changing stressors or environmental exposures.

- **Stress, Movement, and Emotional Well-Being**
  - Chronic stress can tip the microbiome back toward dysbiosis by altering hormone levels and immune responses. Incorporating mindful practices (meditation, light exercise, time in nature) has actually been shown to foster a more stable gut environment.
  - Regular movement—whether strength training, yoga, or moderate cardio—promotes healthy circulation, supports lymphatic drainage, and indirectly benefits gut flora by stabilizing blood sugar and hormone levels.

Tip: "Rebalance" is an ongoing process. Your gut microbes respond to every aspect of your daily routine—food choices, workout regimens, stress levels—so it's worth building healthy, gut-friendly habits you can stick with for the long haul.

A Sample Timeline of the 4 Rs

- **Weeks 1–4 (Remove)**
  - Eliminate processed foods, identify and start treating infections or overgrowths, begin a simplified, anti-inflammatory diet.
- **Weeks 3–8 (Repopulate & Repair Overlap)**
  - Gradually introduce targeted probiotics, fermented foods, prebiotics. Add gut-healing nutrients like glutamine and zinc

carnosine. Watch for improvements or signs of irritation.

- **Weeks 6–12+ (Rebalance)**
    - Transition to a long-term, sustainable diet with personalized fiber intake. Keep stress management routines. Consider retesting if necessary.

Your specific timeline might differ based on test results, symptom severity, and personal response. Some individuals notice dramatic relief within a few weeks; for others, total rebalance can be a months-long journey. The key is consistency and a willingness to tweak your approach as new data (and symptom changes) arise.

Key Takeaways

1. **A Practical Framework**: The four-step approach—Remove, Repopulate, Repair, Rebalance—tackles dysbiosis at its root and builds a robust, health-supporting gut ecosystem.

2. **Start by Clearing Out**: Address infections, eliminate inflammatory foods, and reduce environmental toxins for a "clean slate."

3. **Nourish the Good Bugs**: Probiotics and prebiotics selectively cultivate beneficial strains, while fermented foods offer a gentle, food-based strategy.

4. **Heal the Lining**: L-glutamine, zinc carnosine, and other nutrients rebuild the gut barrier, preventing systemic inflammation.

5. **Maintain and Thrive**: Lifestyle habits—mindful eating, exercise, stress reduction—safeguard your newly balanced microbiome for the long term.

With these steps in hand, you have a tangible plan to address gut imbalances that may have fueled your chronic pain or health struggles for years. Next, we'll walk through common questions, pitfalls, and tips for staying motivated on what can sometimes be a winding but deeply rewarding path to real healing.

10

FAQs, Pitfalls, and Encouragement

—*Addressing Doubts, Avoiding Common Mistakes, and Celebrating Small Wins*

Even with a clear action plan, it's normal to have lingering questions or stumble along the way. As you move from theory to practice—ordering tests, adjusting your diet, trying probiotics—you'll likely encounter moments of uncertainty. This chapter tackles common FAQs, highlights pitfalls to watch for, and offers words of encouragement for staying the course. Healing the gut is not a quick fix; it's a journey that can reshape your relationship with pain, energy, and overall health.

1. Frequently Asked Questions

"Is There Solid Research Backing All This?"

Absolutely. While our understanding of the gut microbiome is still evolving, peer-reviewed studies and clinical trials have repeatedly demonstrated its impact on conditions from irritable bowel syndrome and fibromyalgia to autoimmune disorders and metabolic dysfunction. Journals such as *Gut*, *Cell*, *Nature Microbiology*, and *Microbiome* regularly publish findings on how modulating gut flora can affect systemic inflammation and pain thresholds.

"Do I Have to Take Probiotics Forever?"

No. Many people start with higher doses of targeted probiotics to correct a known imbalance and then scale back once their gut stabilizes. Over time, a balanced diet rich in prebiotic fibers (vegetables, legumes, whole grains) and fermented foods may maintain those benefits naturally. However, some individuals—especially those with recurring infections or autoimmune tendencies—do find that a maintenance dose of probiotics continues to support optimal health.

"What If My Symptoms Flare During the 'Remove' Phase?"

It's common to experience temporary symptom shifts, including mild flare-ups, especially if you're eliminating harmful bacteria or parasites. These microbes can release toxins as they die off (sometimes called a "die-off" or Herxheimer reaction). If discomfort becomes severe, consult your healthcare practitioner for strategies—like reducing antimicrobial doses, staggering probiotics, adding more water intake, or using binders (charcoal, clay) to help clear toxins.

"Can the Wrong Probiotic Make Me Feel Worse?"

Yes. Different strains have different effects, and certain strains might aggravate conditions like SIBO or histamine intolerance. Always pay attention to how you respond when introducing a new supplement or fermented food. If bloating, skin rashes, or other adverse symptoms surge, you might be dealing with an incompatible strain or dose. Work with a practitioner to pinpoint the best approach.

"How Long Before I See Results?"

Timelines vary widely. Some notice better energy or reduced bloating in a few weeks, while deeper issues (autoimmune conditions, chronic pain) can take months to shift. The body needs time to heal from systemic inflammation and rebuild a healthy microbial community. Consistency—both in dietary practices and supplement use—often matters more than speed.

2. Common Pitfalls and How to Avoid Them

Pitfall 1: Self-Diagnosing Without Proper Testing

Relying solely on internet symptom checklists can lead you astray. Comprehensive stool analysis give objective data to guide targeted interventions. Avoid guesswork: invest in proper labs if your symptoms are persistent or severe.

Pitfall 2: Over-Using Antimicrobials

Bombarding your gut with antibiotics or herbal antimicrobials without strategy can disrupt the good bacteria as well as the bad. Work under practitioner guidance, and always support beneficial strains afterward. Overkill can leave you more vulnerable to secondary infections or resistant microbes.

Pitfall 3: Adopting Extreme, Unsustainable Diets

It's tempting to eliminate multiple food groups in hopes of swift relief, but extremely restrictive diets can undermine microbial diversity and lead to nutrient deficiencies. If you must remove certain foods, do so methodically—reintroducing them gradually to assess tolerance. Balancing your gut typically thrives on a diverse array of nutrients.

Pitfall 4: Ignoring Stress and Lifestyle Factors

You can take the best probiotics and eat the cleanest diet, but chronic stress, inadequate sleep, and unresolved emotional issues can still sabotage your progress. The gut–brain–immune axis is real; emotional turmoil can perpetuate dysbiosis just as powerfully as a poor diet. Integrate relaxation techniques, moderate exercise, and healthy sleep hygiene into your routine.

Pitfall 5: Falling for "Miracle Cure" Marketing

The microbiome space is buzzing with hype, which unfortunately attracts questionable products promising overnight transformations. Look for reputable companies that cite peer-reviewed studies, disclose specific strains and CFU counts for probiotics, and encourage comprehensive testing over one-size-fits-all solutions.

3. Celebrating Small Wins

Tracking Progress

Keep a simple journal or use an app to log changes in pain levels, energy, mood, and digestion. Sometimes progress is slow or happens in small increments—a log helps you see that you're gradually improving, even if day-to-day fluctuations can feel frustrating.

Setting Realistic Expectations

Gut healing is a marathon, not a sprint. Applaud each small milestone, whether it's fewer headaches, a better night's sleep, or the ability to enjoy a broader range of foods. Over time, these small wins add up to major improvements in quality of life.

Embracing the Learning Curve

It's normal to make mistakes—like trying a probiotic strain that doesn't agree with you or struggling to cut out certain foods. Each misstep provides data about what your body does or doesn't need. Consider it part of the process rather than a failure.

Sharing Your Story

If you find relief by rebalancing your gut, your story could inspire others who are feeling hopeless. Online communities and support groups can help you stay motivated while also providing practical tips and empathy from people on similar journeys.

4. When to Seek Further Help

While the strategies in this book can offer profound benefits, some conditions require close medical supervision. If you experience severe pain spikes, unexplained weight loss, persistent fever, or other alarming symptoms, consult a healthcare professional promptly. A functional or integrative practitioner who's versed in gut health might be best equipped to guide you, but don't neglect mainstream medical support in emergencies or for necessary diagnostic imaging.

Key Takeaways

1. **Ask the Right Questions**: Proper research and professional guidance boost the odds of success, whether you're dealing with targeted antimicrobials or selecting probiotics.

2. **Avoid Major Pitfalls**: Overusing antimicrobials, jumping on extreme diets, or ignoring stress can derail even the most well-intentioned gut protocol.

3. **Small Wins Matter**: Celebrate improvements as they come—healing is incremental and often requires patience.

4. **Don't Fall for Hype**: Stick to evidence-based products and approaches, and be wary of "silver bullet" marketing claims.

5. **Stay Supported**: Know when to consult professionals and lean on community networks or support groups for lasting motivation.

In the next chapter, we'll dig in deeper into how to avoid scams and make sure you build a solution that's right for you.

11

Beware the Traps: Overdoing Probiotics, Selecting the Wrong Strains, and Staying Scam-Free

—Safeguarding Your Gut-Healing Journey with Informed Choices

Just as the microbiome's importance has surged into the public eye, so too have an array of questionable claims, miracle products, and well-intentioned but overzealous approaches. While certain probiotics can do wonders, choosing them at random—or in high doses without guidance—sometimes backfires, causing more discomfort than relief. Meanwhile, clever marketing and Internet "gurus" may push expensive or risky interventions with minimal scientific backing. In this chapter, we'll highlight the hazards of overdoing it, how to avoid scam pitfalls, and how to course-correct if your gut journey takes a wrong turn.

1. Understanding the Risks of "Probiotic Overload"

Too Much of a Good Thing?

Probiotics have become a modern-day panacea—touted to cure everything from bloating to brain fog. But probiotics are living organisms, and more isn't always better:

- **Excessive Bloating or Distention**
    - Over-supplementation can spark excessive gas production, especially if you already harbor a bacterial overgrowth in the small intestine (SIBO).
    - Certain probiotic strains, like those producing D-lactate, can exacerbate existing gut imbalances for some individuals, leading to cramping or brain fog.
- **Histamine Issues**
    - Some bacteria (e.g., certain Lactobacillus strains) can produce histamine, which may worsen headaches, sinus pressure, or skin rashes for those with histamine intolerance.
- **Competitive Imbalances**
    - Flooding your system with high-dose probiotics could crowd out other beneficial microbes, paradoxically reducing overall diversity.

When in doubt, start low and go slow—introduce one new probiotic at a time, observe how your body reacts, and adjust accordingly.

Matching Strains to Conditions

Different probiotic strains have distinct effects. For instance, while *Saccharomyces boulardii* may help control yeast overgrowth, *Lactobacillus rhamnosus GG* is better known for reducing antibiotic-associated diarrhea. Randomly picking the "strongest" formula might leave you disappointed—or worse, exacerbate symptoms. This is where targeted stool testing and expert input can pay huge dividends.

2. Recognizing Marketing Hype and Scams

Red Flags to Watch For

- **Huge Health Claims Without Evidence**: If a product claims to "cure all autoimmune diseases" or "eliminate chronic pain in days," be skeptical. Legitimate research rarely supports such sweeping guarantees.
- **Proprietary Formulas with Zero Transparency**: Quality probiotic products list strains (e.g., *Lactobacillus acidophilus* La-14), CFU counts, and references to peer-reviewed data. Vague language like "patented blend" with no specifics is a common warning sign.
- **Subscription Pressure**: Some companies auto-enroll you in monthly shipments with high price tags. Make sure to read the fine print and confirm return/refund policies.

Spotting Questionable Providers

Not everyone claiming "gut-health expertise" is properly trained. While functional medicine practitioners and integrative dietitians often specialize in microbiome care, double-check credentials and ask about their approach. Listen for nuances: do they talk about stool analysis, strain specificity, and step-by-step interventions, or just hype a single magic bullet?

3. Course-Correcting When Things Go Wrong

Signs You Need to Pull Back

- **New or Worsening GI Pain**: Severe bloating, diarrhea, or cramping after starting a new supplement can signal an inappropriate strain or dose.
- **Persistent Headaches or Fatigue**: Might be a histamine reaction or an overgrowth of D-lactic acid–producing bacteria.
- **Allergic-like Reactions**: Hives, itching, or respiratory symptoms warrant immediate discontinuation and possibly medical advice.

Practical Steps to Reset

1. **Elimination**: Stop the probiotic or supplement you suspect is causing trouble. Often, symptoms fade within a week or two.
2. **Dietary Simplification**: Scale back on fermentable foods (kombucha, sauerkraut) if you suspect your gut can't handle extra microbes right now.
3. **Retest if Necessary**: If you've had a serious adverse reaction, consider a follow-up stool analysis or consult a practitioner to see if you triggered a secondary imbalance.

4. Avoiding "Natural Cure" Minefields

Beware Unproven Detoxes and Cleanses

From intense parasite cleanses to self-administered antifungal protocols, extreme regimens can disrupt your gut even more severely. Some cleanses incorporate harsh laxatives or questionable substances that irritate the intestinal lining. Unless there's clear evidence of a specific infection (like a proven parasite on a lab test), approach broad-spectrum "cleanses" with caution.

Managing Social Media Trends

Online communities can offer support, but they can also amplify fads. Drastic diets or unconventional supplements might work for a few but backfire for many others. Cross-reference any major advice with scientific literature or a knowledgeable healthcare professional.

5. Staying Empowered

Balancing Healthy Skepticism and Openness

- **Validate**: Check if a new supplement or approach has any peer-reviewed backing.
- **Stay Informed**: Keeping up with credible microbiome research (via sites like PubMed, ScienceDirect) can help you separate real breakthroughs from sensationalized nonsense.
- **Trust Your Body's Signals**: No matter how touted a product is, if you feel markedly worse after introducing it, respect your body's feedback. There's no "universal" cure for everyone's gut.

Positive Use of Probiotics and Gut-Focused Products

Despite the pitfalls, probiotics and gut-health interventions are often game-changers when applied with insight. From targeted strains that quell inflammation to scientifically validated "psychobiotics" that calm anxiety, the key is precision—matching the right intervention to your unique microbial ecosystem.

Key Takeaways

1. **Probiotics Are Powerful—But Not Risk-Free**: Overuse or mismatched strains can worsen bloating, trigger histamine issues, or reduce microbial diversity.

2. **Scams Exploit the Microbiome Buzz**: Avoid miracle-cure promises, vague product labeling, and forced subscription models.

3. **Reset When Necessary**: If a new supplement or protocol clearly backfires, discontinue it and seek professional guidance.

4. **Be Wary of Unproven Cleanses**: Extreme detoxes can do more harm than good without laboratory evidence of specific infections.

5. **Informed and Personalized Is Best**: With well-chosen interventions based on testing and clinical evidence, probiotics and gut therapies can be transformative—just make sure you're using them wisely.

Remember that your gut-health journey is personal. It requires discernment, patience, and a willingness to pivot when something doesn't fit. Still, with the right knowledge and safeguards, you can steer clear of pitfalls and move confidently toward lasting relief.

In our final chapter, we'll bring everything together, with inspiration and guidance for embracing a future that no longer revolves around mysterious pain or health limitations. You've come this far—let's make sure you're equipped to carry this momentum into a pain-free, vibrant future.

12

Closing the Door on "Mysterious" Pain: Embrace Lasting Relief

— Empowering You To Step Confidently Into a Pain-Free Future

You've traveled through a wealth of information—from the scientific underpinnings of the gut–brain–immune axis to real-life stories of transformation, from comprehensive testing options to a step-by-step plan for healing. If there's one overarching message, it's this: **it truly doesn't have to be this way.** Chronic pain, stubborn fatigue, and debilitating flares aren't simply your lot in life. By addressing the microbiome as a root cause, you open up possibilities that conventional medicine often overlooks.

1. Reflecting on the Journey So Far

- **Identifying the Hidden Key**: We began by exploring how an imbalanced gut fuels everything from persistent inflammation to heightened pain signals. This "invisible" factor can remain undetected in countless mainstream tests, yet it can be the missing piece that unlocks a path to relief.
- **Shifting Mindsets**: Embracing a systems-based approach—understanding how the gut, immune system, and nervous system interact—reshapes the way you view pain and chronic illness. Rather than chasing isolated symptoms, you've learned to look upstream and address the root.
- **Comprehensive Strategies**: We covered advanced stool testing, a 4-step gut-restoration blueprint, and crucial tips on choosing the right microbiome tests and probiotics. By marrying scientific insights with a personalized plan, you can transition from trial-and-error frustration to proactive, data-driven care.

2. Your Body's Capacity to Heal

Though it might not feel like it right now, your body has remarkable resilience. Even if you've spent years (or decades) in pain, a battered gut lining can mend, beneficial microbes can recolonize, and immune function can settle into a healthier equilibrium. True, the process can be slow and nonlinear. But countless case studies, clinical trials, and personal testimonies confirm that meaningful recovery is possible.

Reclaiming Hope

Pain and fatigue can cloud your outlook. It's natural to have doubts—especially if you've been told "nothing's wrong" by multiple specialists.

Yet as you've seen in previous chapters, some of the toughest conditions (fibromyalgia, autoimmune disorders, long-standing digestive woes) have responded to microbiome-focused interventions when everything else seemed to fail. Hope becomes practical, not wishful thinking.

3. Creating a Sustainable Future

- **Ongoing Self-Care**: Maintaining a balanced gut isn't a one-and-done affair. Instead, it's woven into daily life: a nutrient-dense diet, mindful stress management, and moderate exercise. The more you integrate these routines, the more your gut health—and overall wellness—stabilizes.
- **Monitoring and Adjustment**: Even after you've achieved a significant reduction in pain or symptoms, staying tuned to your body remains crucial. Over time, hormonal shifts, travel, seasonal changes, or even new life stressors can tug at your microbiome's balance. A periodic "gut check"—through simpler tests or symptom tracking—helps you catch and correct minor imbalances before they escalate.

Celebrating Body-Wide Benefits

Improving your gut often triggers unexpected "bonus" improvements—clearer skin, better mood, sharper mental clarity, and steadier energy levels. By keeping your microbiome resilient, you're also bolstering multiple physiological systems. It's not just about pain relief; it's about vibrant living.

4. Resources and Next Steps

- **Find the Right Practitioner**: If your condition is complex, consider working with a functional or integrative medical professional experienced in intracellular micronutrient testing, interpreting microbiome tests, and crafting individualized protocols.

- **Stay Informed**: Gut-health research evolves rapidly. Check reputable journals, attend webinars by knowledgeable clinicians, and share insights with supportive online communities.
- **Leverage Support**: Chronic illness can isolate you. Look for local or virtual groups where members exchange tips and experiences related to diet changes, supplements, and coping strategies. Being in it together can boost motivation and resilience.

5. Final Encouragement

No single book, test, or supplement "fixes" every ailment—especially if you've been in pain for a long time. But if there's one unwavering truth highlighted across these pages, it's that you **have more control over your health than you might realize**. By targeting the microbiome, you're forging a path that addresses pain at its foundation, paving the way for real, lasting transformation.

It might take time, patience, and more than a few course corrections to fully reclaim your life. Yet each day you choose gut-supportive habits, each moment you invest in understanding how your body responds to certain foods or supplements, and each test you take to gather genuine insights—these all compound into meaningful progress. Small steps indeed can lead to remarkable leaps.

So as you close this final chapter, know that "mysterious" pain doesn't have to remain a mystery. Your gut is central to your well-being, and by nurturing its balance, you're giving your entire body—mind included—permission to heal. You stand at a threshold where chronic suffering no longer dictates your identity or your future. Step confidently into this new chapter of your life—pain-free or, at the very least, pain-reduced and empowered—knowing you have the tools, knowledge, and tenacity to make it a reality.

Key Takeaways

1. **Root-Cause Focus Yields Lasting Relief**: Understanding and caring for the gut can reverse patterns of chronic inflammation and pain that felt incurable.

2. **Resilience Is Possible**: A balanced microbiome fortifies the immune system, nourishes the brain, and paves the way for holistic health.

3. **Stay Curious and Engaged**: Continuous learning about microbiome science and seeking the right support ensure you remain on the path to better health.

4. **Your Future Is Bright**: Mystery pain doesn't have to be your identity. Embrace the forward momentum—your gut can lead the way to a far more vibrant, pain-free life.

Conclusion: Reclaiming Control Over Your Health

— How Your Microbiome Empowers You to Break Free from Chronic Pain

It's often said that the longest journeys begin with a single step. If you've ever felt overwhelmed by pain that no test could explain, or you've encountered the limits of conventional medicine when it comes to "mysterious" symptoms, then consider this book a turning point. Over these chapters, you've come to see that the gut—teeming with trillions of microbes and intimately linked to every facet of your health—is not merely a side note in your healing journey; it's the hidden engine that drives your immunity, energy, and resilience.

Chronic ailments can rob you of hope, creating a spiral of doctor visits, prescription changes, and Internet searches that yield few actionable answers. But as you've read, truly transformative results are possible. By addressing the microbiome directly—through comprehensive testing, targeted interventions, and a renewed focus on lifestyle and stress management—you're stepping into a new framework of health. Rather than feeling powerless, you become a proactive detective, uncovering root causes instead of merely stifling symptoms.

This is not an overnight fix; it's a living process. Expect road bumps. Some treatments might feel right at first, only to need refinement. Certain foods you've eaten for years could suddenly prove irritating, and diets that helped initially might need periodic re-evaluation. Such is the dynamic nature of an ecosystem as complex as your gut. Yet each adjustment, each fresh understanding of how your body responds, brings you one step closer to genuine relief and a far more vibrant life.

Healing is often described as peeling back layers of an onion. Each layer you address—the pathogen that needs clearing, the probiotic strain that flourishes, the nutrient deficiency that repairs your gut lining—reveals deeper opportunities for relief. With each small triumph, your sense of possibility expands. And that new sense of hope is a potent antidote to the fear and fatigue that so often accompany chronic pain.

Above all, remember this: **you have agency. Choice. Autonomy.** If you've been told "it's all in your head" or that you must learn to "just live with it," here is your invitation to press forward. You deserve more than palliative measures or half-answers. Your body is incredibly adaptable. When given the right tools—nutritional, microbial, environmental—it can rebound in ways that even seasoned practitioners find remarkable.

So go ahead: take the next step. Order that comprehensive stool test, try a probiotic strain that specifically addresses your unique imbalance, or make the dietary adjustments that resonate with your body's signals. Seek out practitioners who see the bigger picture. Surround yourself with the kind of supportive community—friends, family, online forums—that will cheer you on.

As you do, know this: **it truly doesn't have to be this way**—the pain, the confusion, the exhaustion. By honoring the central role of your microbiome, you're no longer stuck in a cycle of dead-end treatments. You're on a path of self-discovery and empowerment, moving ever closer to feeling like yourself again—perhaps even better than you can remember.

Take it day by day. Trust in the resilience woven into every cell of your body, and know that you are an active participant in your own healing. Every tweak, every mindful choice, every piece of new data helps guide you toward deeper relief and renewed vitality. The gut is your ally; let it show you just how good life can feel.

Make a Difference with Your Review

You've made it to the end of the book—and the beginning of a more empowered, root-cause approach to your health.

I hope this book helped you understand how deeply your gut impacts your energy, mood, immunity, and pain—and gave you tools to finally get unstuck when nothing else has worked.

If it brought you clarity, direction, or hope, I have one small request: would you consider helping others by taking one minute to leave a review?

Why Your Review Matters—It's Simple, Fast, and Makes an Impact

Most people searching for answers are just like you were—exhausted and frustrated, feeling stuck, unsure who to trust, and desperate for real relief. Your review could help:

- One more person connect their gut health to their fatigue, anxiety, or autoimmune flares
- One more patient realize they're not crazy for feeling awful with "normal" labs
- One more reader discover that bloating, migraines, joint pain, or brain fog aren't random—they're clues
- One more person take action and achieve real healing, not just symptom suppression

Your story might be the spark that helps someone else start healing from the inside out.

How to Leave a Review

It only takes one or two sentences—share what resonated with you the most. To leave your review, please scan the QR code below or visit:
https://www.amazon.com/review/review-your-purchases/?asin=B0F27C
7L4W

Thank You for Paying It Forward

I hope this book gave you answers and direction—and I'm grateful for your voice helping others discover the power of healing the gut, one reader at a time.

With deep gratitude,
Keryn Gold, PhD, MBA

Author, *Gut Health Breakthrough*
LeadWithGold.com

Appendix: Therapeutic Doses of Absorbable Micronutrients

— How to Support Gut Health With Vitamins & Minerals Your Body Can Actually Use

Not all vitamins and minerals absorb at the same rate. Some forms are **easily used by your body**, while others **pass through your digestive system without really doing anything.**

Also, dosage matters.

- If you take **too little** of a nutrient, it may not be enough to **fix a deficiency**.
- If you take **too much**, it can **build up in your system and cause new problems.**
- Some nutrients **require a balance with other nutrients**—tak-

ing too much of one can throw off another.

This is why **just knowing what to take isn't enough—you have to take the right amount in the right way.**

Intracellular Vitamins, Minerals, Amino Acids, Antioxidants, & Nutrients

Here is an excerpt from one of my other books, *The Root Cause of Your Symptoms, Uncovered,* where we outline key micronutrients and the far-reaching effects they have on the body, including how they relate to gut health, both as a cause and consequence. For each, we share the best, most absorbable sources to address intracellular deficiency (functional intracellular micronutrient deficiencies can be tested by Genova Biosciences or Spectracell, among others), and highlight the **therapeutic dose** for each micronutrient. Please note that therapeutic doses often exceed the recommended daily allowances (RDAs) and should only be taken under medical supervision, if you're sure you have a deficiency.

Vitamin A

- **Role**: Helps your eyes see clearly, especially at night, and keeps your skin healthy and strong.
- **Deficiency symptoms:** Night blindness, dry skin, weakened immunity, corneal drying (keratomalacia).
- **Most absorbable form:** Retinyl palmitate or retinol.
- **Least absorbable form:** Beta-carotene from food (requires conversion).
- **RDA:** 900 mcg RAE (men), 700 mcg RAE (women).

- **Top food sources:**
  - Sweet potato (1 medium): ~1,096 mcg RAE.
  - Carrots (1/2 cup cooked): ~671 mcg RAE.
  - Spinach (1/2 cup cooked): ~573 mcg RAE.
- **Therapeutic dose:** 10,000–25,000 IU/day.
- **Toxic dose:** >25,000 IU/day chronically or >300,000 IU acutely.
- **Overdose effects:** Liver damage, intracranial hypertension, birth defects in pregnancy.

Vitamin B1 (Thiamin)

- **Role**: Turns food into energy to help your brain and muscles work properly.
- **Deficiency symptoms:** Fatigue, irritability, memory loss, beriberi (wet: heart failure; dry: nerve damage), Wernicke-Korsakoff syndrome.
- **Most absorbable form:** Thiamin mononitrate or benfotiamine.
- **Least absorbable form:** Thiamin hydrochloride in low-quality supplements.
- **RDA:** 1.2 mg (men), 1.1 mg (women).
- **Top food sources:**
  - Pork chop (3 oz): ~0.81 mg.
  - Black beans (1 cup cooked): ~0.42 mg.

  - Fortified cereal (1 cup): ~1.5 mg.

- **Therapeutic dose:** 50–100 mg/day for deficiency or neuropathy.
- **Toxic dose:** No established toxic dose; excess is peed out.

Vitamin B2 (Riboflavin)

- **Role**: Helps your body use food to make energy and keeps your eyes and skin healthy.
- **Deficiency symptoms:** Cracked lips, sore throat, inflamed tongue (glossitis), sensitivity to light, skin rashes.
- **Most absorbable form:** Riboflavin-5'-phosphate.
- **Least absorbable form:** Free riboflavin in low-quality supplements.
- **RDA:** 1.3 mg (men), 1.1 mg (women).
- **Top food sources:**
  - Beef liver (3 oz): ~3 mg.
  - Yogurt (1 cup plain): ~0.45 mg.
  - Almonds (1 oz): ~0.23 mg.
- **Therapeutic dose:** 25–100 mg/day for migraines or deficiency.
- **Toxic dose:** No established toxic dose; excess excreted in urine.

Vitamin B3 (Niacin)

- **Role**: Helps turn food into energy, keeps your skin healthy, and helps nerves work well.

- **Deficiency symptoms:** Pellagra—diarrhea, dermatitis, dementia; fatigue; depression; skin irritation.
- **Most absorbable form:** Nicotinamide or niacinamide (non-flushing).
- **Least absorbable form:** Inositol hexanicotinate ("no-flush" niacin).
- **RDA:** 16 mg NE (men), 14 mg NE (women).
- **Top food sources:**
  - Chicken breast (3 oz cooked): ~10.3 mg NE.
  - Tuna (3 oz cooked): ~11 mg NE.
  - Fortified cereal (1 cup): ~20–27 mg NE.
- **Therapeutic dose:** 500–2000 mg/day for cholesterol management or deficiency.
- **Toxic dose:** >2000 mg/day can cause liver damage and flushing effects.
- **Overdose effects:** Skin flushing, liver toxicity.

Vitamin B5 (Pantothenic Acid)

- **Role**: Helps turn the food you eat into energy and helps build important body chemicals.
- **Deficiency symptoms:** Fatigue, numbness/burning feet syndrome, irritability.

- **Most absorbable form:** Calcium pantothenate or pantethine.
- **Least absorbable form:** Free pantothenic acid in low-quality supplements.
- **AI (Adequate Intake):** 5 mg/day.
- **Top food sources:**
  - Shiitake mushrooms (1/2 cup cooked): ~2.6 mg.
  - Avocado (1/2 fruit): ~1 mg.
  - Sunflower seeds (1 oz): ~2.2 mg.
- **Therapeutic dose:** 500–1000 mg/day for adrenal support or acne treatment.
- **Toxic dose:** >10 g/day can cause diarrhea and gastrointestinal distress.

Vitamin B6 (Pyridoxine)

- **Role**: Helps your brain communicate clearly, helps make red blood cells, and helps break down proteins.
- **Deficiency symptoms:** Anemia, depression, confusion, weakened immune system, dermatitis, cracked and sore lips, inflamed tongue.
- **Most absorbable form**: Pyridoxal-5'-phosphate (P5P).
- **Least absorbable form**: Pyridoxine hydrochloride in low-quality supplements.
- **RDA**: 1.3-1.7 mg/day for adults.

- **Top food sources**: Chickpeas (1 cup cooked): ~1.1 mg, Tuna (3 oz): ~0.9 mg, Potato (1 medium): ~0.4 mg.
- **Therapeutic dose**: 50-200 mg/day for carpal tunnel syndrome or morning sickness.
- **Toxic dose**: >200 mg/day long-term can cause neuropathy.
- **Overdose effects**: Sensory neuropathy, ataxia.

Vitamin B12 (Cobalamin)

- **Role**: Helps make healthy blood cells and keeps your brain and nerves working properly.
- **Deficiency symptoms**: Fatigue, weakness, constipation, loss of appetite, weight loss, numbness and tingling in hands and feet, difficulty maintaining balance, depression, confusion, poor memory, soreness of the mouth or tongue.
- **Most absorbable form**: Methylcobalamin or adenosylcobalamin.
- **Least absorbable form**: Cyanocobalamin for those with certain genetic mutations.
- **RDA**: 2.4 mcg/day for adults.
- **Top food sources**: Clams (3 oz): ~84 mcg, Beef liver (3 oz): ~70 mcg, Fortified nutritional yeast (1 tbsp): ~2.4 mcg.
- **Therapeutic dose**: 1000-5000 mcg/day for deficiency or pernicious anemia.
- **Toxic dose**: No known toxicity from oral intake.

- **Overdose effects**: No known adverse effects from high oral doses.

Vitamin C (Ascorbic Acid)

- **Role**: Protects you from getting sick, helps cuts heal faster, and helps keep teeth and gums healthy.
- **Deficiency symptoms**: Fatigue, weakness, irritability, weight loss, muscle and joint pains, easy bruising, dry skin, splitting hair, swollen and discolored gums, sudden gum bleeding, poor wound healing, weakened immunity.
- **Most absorbable form**: Liposomal vitamin C.
- **Least absorbable form**: Ascorbic acid in high doses (due to saturation of absorption).
- **RDA**: 90 mg/day (men), 75 mg/day (women).
- **Top food sources**: Red bell pepper (1/2 cup raw): ~95 mg, Orange (1 medium): ~70 mg, Kiwifruit (1 medium): ~64 mg.
- **Therapeutic dose**: 500-2000 mg/day for immune support or antioxidant benefits.
- **Toxic dose**: >2000 mg/day may cause gastrointestinal distress.
- **Overdose effects**: Diarrhea, nausea, abdominal cramps, kidney stones in susceptible individuals.

Vitamin D

- **Role**: Helps your bones grow strong by helping your body use calcium from food.

- **Deficiency symptoms**: Bone pain, muscle weakness, increased risk of fractures, fatigue, depression.
- **Most absorbable form**: Vitamin D3 (cholecalciferol).
- **Least absorbable form**: Vitamin D2 (ergocalciferol).
- **RDA**: 600-800 IU/day for adults.
- **Top food sources**: Salmon (3 oz cooked): ~570 IU, Fortified milk (1 cup): ~120 IU, Egg yolk (1 large): ~40 IU.
- **Therapeutic dose**: 2000-5000 IU/day for deficiency or bone health.
- **Toxic dose**: >10,000 IU/day long-term can lead to hypercalcemia.
- **Overdose effects**: Hypercalcemia, kidney stones, calcification of soft tissues.

Vitamin E

- **Role**: Protects your cells from damage, keeping your heart healthy and skin smooth.
- **Deficiency symptoms**: Nerve and muscle damage, loss of body movement control, muscle weakness, vision problems.
- **Most absorbable form**: Mixed tocopherols and tocotrienols.
- **Least absorbable form**: Synthetic dl-alpha-tocopherol.
- **RDA**: 15 mg/day (22.4 IU) for adults.
- **Top food sources**: Sunflower seeds (1 oz): ~7.4 mg, Almonds (1 oz): ~7.3 mg, Hazelnuts (1 oz): ~4.3 mg.

- **Therapeutic dose**: 400-800 IU/day for antioxidant support or skin health.
- **Toxic dose**: >1000 mg/day of alpha-tocopherol can increase bleeding risk.
- **Overdose effects**: Increased risk of bleeding, especially when combined with blood thinners.

Vitamin K

- **Role**: Helps stop bleeding when you get a cut by helping blood clot quickly.
- **Deficiency symptoms**: Easy bruising, excessive bleeding, slow blood clotting, osteoporosis.
- **Most absorbable form**: Vitamin K2 (MK-7).
- **Least absorbable form**: Vitamin K1 (phylloquinone) from plant sources.
- **AI (Adequate Intake)**: 120 mcg/day (men), 90 mcg/day (women).
- **Top food sources**: Kale (1/2 cup cooked): ~531 mcg, Spinach (1/2 cup cooked): ~444 mcg, Brussels sprouts (1/2 cup cooked): ~109 mcg.
- **Therapeutic dose**: 100-300 mcg/day as Vitamin K2 for bone and cardiovascular health.
- **Toxic dose**: No known toxicity from oral intake.
- **Overdose effects**: Can interfere with blood-thinning medications.

FOLATE (VITAMIN B9)

- **Role**: Helps your body make new cells, especially important for growing children.
- **Deficiency symptoms**: Fatigue, weakness, irritability, headache, heart palpitations, shortness of breath, open sores on the tongue and inside the mouth, changes in skin, hair, or fingernail color, growth problems.
- **Most absorbable form**: Methylfolate (L-5-MTHF).
- **Least absorbable form**: Folic acid for those with MTHFR gene mutations.
- **RDA**: 400 mcg DFE/day for adults.
- **Top food sources**: Beef liver (3 oz): ~215 mcg DFE, Spinach (1/2 cup cooked): ~131 mcg DFE, Black-eyed peas (1/2 cup cooked): ~105 mcg DFE.
- **Therapeutic dose**: 400-1000 mcg/day as methylfolate for various health conditions.
- **Toxic dose**: No known toxicity, but high doses can mask B12 deficiency.
- **Overdose effects**: May exacerbate symptoms in some people with anxiety or sleep issues.

BIOTIN (VITAMIN B7)

- **Role**: Helps turn food into energy and keeps your hair, skin, and nails strong.

- **Deficiency symptoms**: Hair loss, scaly red rash around eyes, nose, mouth, and genitals, depression, lethargy, hallucinations, numbness and tingling in extremities.
- **Most absorbable form**: D-biotin.
- **Least absorbable form**: No significant difference in forms.
- **AI (Adequate Intake)**: 30 mcg/day for adults.
- **Top food sources**: Egg yolk (1 large): ~10 mcg, Salmon (3 oz cooked): ~5 mcg, Sunflower seeds (1/4 cup): ~2.6 mcg.
- **Therapeutic dose**: 2-5 mg/day for hair, skin, and nail health.
- **Toxic dose**: No known toxicity from oral intake.
- **Overdose effects**: May interfere with certain lab tests, including thyroid function tests.

Calcium

- **Role**: Builds strong bones and teeth, helps muscles move, nerves send messages, and blood clot when you're hurt.
- **Deficiency symptoms**: Muscle cramps, numbness and tingling in fingers, abnormal heart rhythms, bone fractures.
- **Most absorbable form**: Calcium citrate.
- **Least absorbable form**: Calcium carbonate (especially when taken without food).
- **RDA**: 1000-1200 mg/day for adults.
- **Top food sources**: Yogurt (1 cup plain): ~415 mg, Sardines (3 oz

with bones): ~325 mg, Milk (1 cup): ~300 mg.

- **Therapeutic dose**: 1000-1500 mg/day for bone health or deficiency.
- **Toxic dose**: >2500 mg/day can lead to hypercalcemia.
- **Overdose effects**: Kidney stones, constipation, interference with absorption of other minerals.

Magnesium

- **Role**: Helps muscles relax after they move, keeps bones strong, helps nerves communicate clearly, and helps your heart beat normally.
- **Deficiency symptoms**: Muscle cramps, fatigue, irregular heartbeat, osteoporosis, high blood pressure, anxiety, depression.
- **Most absorbable form**: Magnesium glycinate or magnesium threonate.
- **Least absorbable form**: Magnesium oxide.
- **RDA**: 400-420 mg/day (men), 310-320 mg/day (women).
- **Top food sources**: Pumpkin seeds (1 oz): ~156 mg, Spinach (1/2 cup cooked): ~78 mg, Black beans (1/2 cup cooked): ~60 mg.
- **Therapeutic dose**: 300-600 mg/day for various health conditions.
- **Toxic dose**: >5000 mg/day from supplements can cause diarrhea and nausea.
- **Overdose effects**: Diarrhea, nausea, abdominal cramping, irreg-

ular heartbeat in severe cases.

Manganese

- **Role**: Helps bones grow properly and helps the body turn food into energy.
- **Deficiency symptoms**: Poor bone growth, joint pain, impaired glucose metabolism, infertility, skin rashes
- **Most absorbable form**: Manganese glycinate or gluconate
- **Least absorbable form**: Manganese sulfate or oxide
- **AI (Adequate Intake)**: Men 2.3 mg/day, Women 1.8 mg/day
- **Top food sources**: Pineapple (½ cup raw): ~0.8 mg, Pecans (1 oz): ~1.3 mg, Brown rice (½ cup cooked): ~1.1 mg
- **Therapeutic dose**: 5–10 mg/day for bone and joint health
- **Toxic dose**: >11 mg/day chronically can cause neurological issues
- **Overdose effects**: Neurological symptoms similar to Parkinson's disease (tremors, rigidity)

Copper

- **Role**: Helps form red blood cells that carry oxygen around the body; also keeps nerves healthy.
- **Deficiency symptoms**: Fatigue, anemia, poor immunity, osteoporosis, pale skin/hair graying prematurely
- **Most absorbable form**: Copper glycinate or gluconate

- **Least absorbable form**: Copper oxide or sulfate
- **RDA**: Adults 900 mcg/day
- **Top food sources**: Beef liver (3 oz): ~12 mg, Oysters (3 oz): ~4.8 mg, Cashews (1 oz): ~0.6 mg
- **Therapeutic dose**: 1–3 mg/day for deficiency or anemia
- **Toxic dose**: >10 mg/day chronically can cause liver damage
- **Overdose effects**: Liver and kidney damage, nausea, vomiting

Chromium

- **Role**: Helps keep blood sugar steady so you have balanced energy throughout the day.
- **Deficiency symptoms**: Poor glucose control, insulin resistance, fatigue, anxiety, increased cholesterol levels
- **Most absorbable form**: Chromium picolinate or chromium polynicotinate
- **Least absorbable form**: Chromium chloride or oxide
- **AI**: Men 35 mcg/day; Women 25 mcg/day
- **Top food sources**: Broccoli (½ cup cooked): ~11 mcg, Grape juice (1 cup): ~8 mcg, Turkey breast (3 oz): ~2 mcg
- **Therapeutic dose**: 200–1000 mcg/day for blood sugar regulation and insulin sensitivity
- **Toxic dose**: >1200 mcg/day chronically may be harmful to kidneys/liver

- **Overdose effects**: Kidney/liver damage at very high doses

Selenium

- **Role**: Protects cells from damage, helps keep your immune system strong so you don't get sick easily, and helps the thyroid gland control how fast you grow.
- **Deficiency symptoms**: Fatigue, thyroid dysfunction, poor immunity, infertility in men and women, hair loss
- **Most absorbable form**: Selenomethionine or selenium glycinate chelate
- **Least absorbable form**: Sodium selenite or selenate (inorganic forms)
- **RDA**: Adults 55 mcg/day
- **Top food sources**: Brazil nuts (1 nut): ~68–91 mcg; Tuna (3 oz cooked): ~92 mcg; Halibut (3 oz cooked): ~47 mcg
- **Therapeutic dose**: 100–200 mcg/day for thyroid health and antioxidant support
- **Toxic dose**: >400–600 mcg/day chronically can cause toxicity (selenosis)
- **Overdose effects**: Hair loss, brittle nails, garlic breath odor

Zinc

- **Role**: Keeps your immune system strong to fight germs; helps wounds heal faster; important for taste and smell.

- **Deficiency symptoms**: Poor wound healing, weakened immunity, loss of taste/smell, hair loss/thinning hair
- **Most absorbable form**: Zinc picolinate or zinc bisglycinate
- **Least absorbable form**: Zinc oxide
- **RDA**: Men 11 mg/day; Women 8 mg/day
- **Top food sources**: Oysters (3 oz): ~74 mg; Beef (3 oz cooked): ~5.3 mg; Pumpkin seeds (¼ cup): ~2.9 mg
- **Therapeutic dose**: 15–30 mg/day for immune support and wound healing
- **Toxic dose**: >40–50 mg/day chronically can cause copper deficiency
- **Overdose effects**: Nausea/vomiting; copper deficiency leading to anemia

Alpha Lipoic Acid (ALA)

- **Role**: Protects cells from damage; helps turn sugar into energy; keeps nerves healthy so you can feel things properly.
- **Deficiency symptoms**: Neuropathy symptoms in diabetics; fatigue; oxidative stress signs
- **Most absorbable form**: R-alpha-lipoic acid
- **Least absorbable form**: Synthetic racemic alpha-lipoic acid
- **RDA/AI** not established
- **Top food sources** (small amounts only): Beef liver (~5–10

mg/serving), spinach/broccoli (<1 mg/serving)

- **Therapeutic dose**: 300–600 mg/day for neuropathy or antioxidant support
- **Toxic dose**: >1800–2400 mg/day may cause side effects
- **Overdose effects**: Nausea/vomiting; hypoglycemia; dizziness

Coenzyme Q10 (CoQ10)

- **Role**: Gives cells energy so they can do their jobs; especially important for keeping the heart beating strongly.
- **Deficiency symptoms**: Fatigue; muscle weakness/pain; heart problems; high blood pressure
- **Most absorbable form**: Ubiquinol (reduced CoQ10)
- **Least absorbable form**: Ubiquinone in powder/tablet forms without fat/oil base
- **RDA/**AI not established
- **Top food sources** (small amounts only): Organ meats (~2–4 mg/serving), fatty fish (~2–3 mg/serving)
- **Therapeutic dose**: 100–300 mg/day for cardiovascular health and energy production
- **Toxic dose not established:** generally safe up to 1200 mg/day
- **Overdose effects** rare but may include digestive upset

Cysteine/N-Acetyl Cysteine (NAC)

- **Role**: Helps protect lungs; makes a special chemical called glutathione that cleans up harmful things inside cells.
- **Deficiency symptoms**: Low glutathione levels; poor detoxification ability; frequent infections
- **Most absorbable form**: N-Acetyl cysteine (NAC) supplement form
- **Least absorbable form** not applicable as NAC is standard supplemental form
- **RDA**/AI not established
- **Top food sources** (~100–300mg/serving): Chicken/turkey breast (~200mg), eggs (~150mg), yogurt (~100mg)
- **Therapeutic dose** NAC supplement form only—500–1500mg daily for antioxidant/detox support & respiratory health
- **Toxic dose**: >7 grams daily can cause toxicity/side effects
- **Overdose effects** nausea/vomiting/dizziness

Glutathione

- **Role**: Cleans up waste inside cells; protects them from damage; helps keep you healthy by fighting germs and toxins.
- **Deficiency symptoms**: fatigue; oxidative stress signs; weakened immune system; poor detoxification ability
- **Most absorbable form**: liposomal glutathione supplement or

intravenous glutathione therapy

- **Least absorbable form**: oral non-liposomal glutathione supplements due to poor absorption/breakdown in gut
- **RDA**/AI not established
- **Top food sources**: Avocado (~27mg), asparagus (~28mg/cup), spinach (~11mg/cup cooked)
- **Therapeutic dose**: liposomal glutathione supplement—250–1000mg daily
- **Toxic dose**: no known toxicity from oral intake

CHOLINE

- **Role**: Helps brain cells communicate clearly so you can think well; also protects liver health by removing fat buildup.
- **Deficiency symptoms:** fatty liver disease; memory problems/cognitive decline; muscle weakness/pain
- **Most absorbable form**: Alpha-GPC or Citicoline supplements
- **Least absorbable form**: Choline bitartrate supplements
- **AI:** men 550mg/day women 425mg/day
- **Top foods**: Beef liver (~356mg/3oz), eggs (~147mg per egg), chicken breast (~72mg per serving)
- **Therapeutic dose**: 500–2000mg daily for brain health/fatty liver disease
- **Toxic dose**: >3500mg daily chronically may cause side effects

- **Overdose effects:** fishy body odor/nausea/vomiting

Inositol

- **Role**: Keeps mood balanced so you feel calm and happy; also helps cells talk to each other clearly.
- **Deficiency symptoms**: anxiety/depression/mood swings/panic attacks
- **Most absorbable form:** Myo-inositol supplement powder
- **Least absorbable form**: no significant differences known
- **No RDA established** – therapeutic doses range from 2–12 grams daily for mood disorders/hormonal balance
- **Food sources**: citrus fruits/grains/nuts (~50–100mg per serving) small amounts only
- **No known toxic dose** or overdose effects.

Carnitine

- **Role**: Turns fat into energy so muscles have enough power to move; helps keep the heart healthy.
- **Deficiency symptoms**: fatigue/muscle weakness/impaired fat metabolism
- **Most absorbable form**: Acetyl-L-carnitine supplement
- **Least absorbable form**: D-carnitine synthetic forms
- **No RDA established** – therapeutic doses range from

500–2000mg daily for energy production/cognitive support

- **Food sources**: beef (~81mg/3oz), fish/chicken (~5–10mg per serving) small amounts only
- **No known toxic dose** or overdose effects.

Asparagine

- **What it does in your body:** Helps your body make proteins, keeps your brain and nerves healthy, helps cells survive when stressed or low on nutrients, and helps balance other amino acids in your cells
- **What deficiency feels like (symptoms):** Tiredness, confusion, weakened immune system, trouble thinking clearly, poor cell function
- **Most absorbable form:** L-asparagine (natural amino acid form)
- **Least absorbable form:** D-asparagine (unnatural form, poorly utilized by the body)
- **Recommended daily value (RDA/AI):** No official RDA established; typically obtained sufficiently from diet.
- **Top 3 food sources and amounts per serving:**
    - Asparagus (~500 mg per cup cooked)
    - Potatoes (~400 mg per medium potato)
    - Eggs (~300 mg per large egg)
- **Therapeutic dose:** Typically not supplemented individually; dietary intake sufficient. If used therapeutically under medical su-

pervision: ~500–1000 mg/day.

- **Toxic dose:** No known toxic dose from dietary sources or normal supplementation.
- **Overdose effects:** No known harmful effects from normal dietary intake; extremely high unnatural supplementation could theoretically disrupt amino acid balance.

Glutamine

- **What it does in your body:** Helps build proteins, provides energy to cells (especially intestinal and immune cells), removes waste products like ammonia from your body, helps maintain acid-base balance in kidneys, supports immune system function, and helps heal your gut lining
- **What deficiency feels like (symptoms):** Weak immune system, frequent infections, digestive problems, muscle weakness or soreness, fatigue, slow recovery after illness or injury
- **Most absorbable form:** L-glutamine powder or capsules
- **Least absorbable form:** D-glutamine (unnatural form)
- **Recommended daily value (RDA/AI):** No official RDA established; typical dietary intake ~3–6 grams/day.
- **Top 3 food sources and amounts per serving:**
    - Beef (~1.2 grams per 3 oz serving)
    - Chicken (~1 gram per 3 oz serving)
    - Eggs (~0.6 grams per large egg)

al health. Integrative Medicine: A Clinician's Journal, 8.

A. (2012). Leaky gut and autoimmune dis- nical Reviews in Allergy & Immunology, 42(1), s://doi.org/10.1007/s12016-011-8291-x

A., Hyde, E., Sangwan, N., Gilbert, J. A., & Knight, Migraine patients exhibit distinct oral and gut micro- Systems, 1(5), e00105-16. https://doi.org/10.1128/mSys- -16

ing, X., Shen, Y., Lyon, C. J., & Wang, X. (2023). Gut in autoimmune diseases. Frontiers in Immunology, 13, ttps://doi.org/10.3389/fimmu.2022.1003684

A., Tillisch, K., & Gupta, A. (2015). Gut/brain axis nicrobiota. Journal of Clinical Investigation, 125(3), ttps://doi.org/10.1172/JCI76304

G. M., Johnson, A. C., O'Mahony, S. M., Dinan, T. G., d-Van Meerveld, B., & Cryan, J. F. (2016). Stress and biota-gut-brain axis in visceral pain: relevance to irrita- syndrome. CNS Neuroscience & Therapeutics, 22(2), ttps://doi.org/10.1111/cns.12490

rby, J., Reilly, C. M., & Luo, X. M. (2017). Leaky gut as a al for autoimmune diseases. Frontiers in Immunology, 8, //doi.org/10.3389/fimmu.2017.00598

ang, H., & Luo, X. M. (2015). SLE: Another autoimmune fluenced by microbes and diet? Frontiers in Immunology, s://doi.org/10.3389/fimmu.2015.00608

S. M., Clarke, G., Borre, Y. E., Dinan, T. G., J. F. (2015). Serotonin, tryptophan metabolism and

- **Therapeutic dose:** 5–30 grams/day (for gut health, immune support, muscle recovery)
- **Toxic dose:** >40 grams/day chronically may cause side effects
- **Overdose effects:** Digestive upset, nausea, dizziness; very high doses may worsen kidney or liver problems

Serine

- **What it does in your body:** Helps build proteins needed for muscles and nerves to work well; important for brain function; helps make other important molecules like DNA and RNA; supports healthy cell membranes and nerve signaling
- **What deficiency feels like (symptoms):** Neurological symptoms such as poor coordination or seizures (rare), cognitive impairment or confusion, muscle weakness
- **Most absorbable form:** L-serine supplement form.
- **Least absorbable form:** D-serine (less utilized by the body).
- **Recommended daily value (RDA/AI):** No official RDA established; typical dietary intake ~1–3 grams/day.
- **Top 3 food sources and amounts per serving:**
  - Soybeans (~2 grams per cup cooked)
  - Eggs (~0.5 grams per large egg)
  - Lentils (~0.4 grams per cup cooked)
- **Therapeutic dose:** ~500 mg–2 grams/day for neurological support or cognitive health.

- **Toxic dose:** No known toxic dose from normal dietary intake or typical supplementation.
- **Overdose effects:** Generally safe; extremely high doses could cause mild digestive upset.

These nutrients, vitamins, minerals, antioxidants, and amino acids work together every day to keep you healthy, strong, growing well, thinking clearly, feeling good emotionally, healing quickly when you're hurt or sick, and giving you enough energy to play, learn, and explore. But when any one of them breaks down or isn't being absorbed into cells or working correctly, it can have cascading effects that lead to multiple symptoms.

Remember to be careful with supplementation – it's possible to take too much for your specific circumstance, which can be dangerous, so it's important to consult with a healthcare professional before starting any new supplement regimen, as individual needs may vary.

For more information, please check out a copy of *The Root Cause of Your Symptoms, Uncovered* or visit LeadWithGold.com/heal for additional free resources and downloads.

REFEREN

Allen, A. P., Hutch, W., Borr
Temko, A., Boylan, G., & Cry
terium longum 1714 as a psychobi
An exploratory study. Journal of Psyc
612–618. https://doi.org/10.1016/j.jpsy

Bischoff, S. C., Barbara, G., Buu
Schulzke, J. D., Serino, M., Tilg,
J. M. (2014). Intestinal permeabil
ease prevention and therapy. BMC
189. https://doi.org/10.1186/s12876-01

Cani, P. D., Bibiloni, R., Knauf, C.,
Delzenne, N. M., & Burcelin, R. (
crobiota control metabolic endotoxen
high-fat diet–induced obesity and diab
1470–1481. https://doi.org/10.2337/dt

Cleveland Clinic. (n.d.). Dysbiosis.
from https://my.clevelandclinic.org/hea

Dolan, K. E., Finley, H. J., Burns, C. M.,
Parker, E. C., Pizano, J. M., Williamson,
Probiotics and disease: A comprehensive

neurolo
15(5), 46

Fasano,
eases. C
71-78. ht

Gonzale
R. (2016
biomes.
tems.001

Guo, Y.,
microbio
1003684.

Mayer, E
and the
926–938.

Moloney,
Greenwo
the micr
ble bowe
102–117.

Mu, Q.,
danger si
598. http

Mu, Q., Z
disorder i
6, 608. ht

O'Mahon
& Cryan

the brain-gut-microbiome axis. Behavioural Brain Research, 277, 32–48. https://doi.org/10.1016/j.bbr.2014.07.027

Peng, J., Xiao, X., Hu, M., & Zhang, X. (2018). Interaction between gut microbiome and cardiovascular disease. Life Sciences, 214, 153-157. https://doi.org/10.1016/j.lfs.2018.10.063

Quince, C., Walker, A. W., Simpson, J. T., Loman, N. J., & Segata, N. (2017). Shotgun metagenomics, from sampling to analysis. Nature Biotechnology, 35(9), 833–844. https://doi.org/10.1038/nbt.3935

Resnick, C., Kechichian, E., Safi, R., Awada, H., Maalouf, D., Khoury, R., Kechichian, J., & Tomb, R. (2022). Leaky gut and autoimmune diseases: From bench to bedside. Frontiers in Immunology, 13, 860565. https://doi.org/10.3389/fimmu.2022.860565

Sampson, T. R., Debelius, J. W., Thron, T., Janssen, S., Shastri, G. G., Ilhan, Z. E., ... Mazmanian, S. K. (2016). Gut microbiota regulate motor deficits and neuroinflammation in a model of Parkinson's disease. Cell, 167(6), 1469–1480.e12. https://doi.org/10.1016/j.cell.2016.11.018

Sánchez, B., Delgado, S., Blanco-Míguez, A., Lourenço, A., Gueimonde, M., & Margolles, A. (2017). Probiotics, gut microbiota, and their influence on host health and disease. Molecular Nutrition & Food Research, 61(1), 1600240. https://doi.org/10.1002/mnfr.201600240

Scher, J. U., Sczesnak, A., Longman, R. S., Segata, N., Ubeda, C., Bielski, C., ... Littman, D. R. (2013). Expansion of intestinal Prevotella copri correlates with enhanced susceptibility to arthritis. eLife, 2, e01202. https://doi.org/10.7554/eLife.01202

Strandwitz, P. (2018). Neurotransmitter modulation by the gut microbiota. Current Opinion in Microbiology, 24, 41–45. https://doi.org/10.1016/j.mib.2018.07.002

Sturgeon, C., & Fasano, A. (2016). Zonulin, a regulator of epithelial and endothelial barrier functions, and its involvement in chronic inflammatory diseases. Tissue Barriers, 4(4), e1251384. https://doi.org/10.1080/21688370.2016.1251384

Turnbaugh, P. J., Ridaura, V. K., Faith, J. J., Rey, F. E., Knight, R., & Gordon, J. I. (2021). The effect of gut microbiota on host metabolism: New insights from metagenomics. Cell, 184(8), 1970–1986. https://doi.org/10.1016/j.cell.2021.02.056

Vaghef-Mehrabany, E., Alipour, B., Homayouni-Rad, A., Sharif, S. K., Asghari-Jafarabadi, M., & Zavvari, S. (2014). Probiotic supplementation improves inflammatory status in patients with rheumatoid arthritis. Nutrition, 30(4), 430–435. https://doi.org/10.1016/j.nut.2013.09.007

Zhang, H., Sparks, J. B., Karyala, S. V., Settlage, R., & Luo, X. M. (2015). A refocused immune system tolerates endogenous microbiota. Science, 347(6226), 865–869. https://doi.org/10.1126/science.aaa7032

Made in the USA
Monee, IL
04 November 2026

67378713R00069